THE PATIENT RECRUITMENT CONUNDRUM

ROSS JACKSON

Copyright © Ross Jackson 2023

All Rights Reserved. No part of this publication may be reproduced, stored in a retrieval system, or transmitted in any form, or by any means, electronic, mechanical, photocopying, recording or otherwise without the prior permission in writing of the copyright holders, nor be otherwise circulated in any form or binding or cover other than in which it is published and without a similar condition being imposed on the subsequent publisher.

This is a work of fiction. Any names or characters, businesses or places, events or incidents, are fictitious. Any resemblance to actual persons, living or dead, or actual events is purely coincidental.

Contents

Preface i

Chapter One – The Invitation. 1

Chapter Two – Flight into the Unknown 5

Chapter Three – Hotel Homecoming. 9

Chapter Four – Wexford's World of Wealth 13

Chapter Five – Sarcastic Sidekick 19

Chapter Six – The Journey Begins 25

Chapter Seven – The Research Site. 29

Chapter Eight – Debrief and Download. 41

Chapter Nine – The CRO 47

Chapter Ten – A Pub Lunch. 55

Chapter Eleven – The Patient Advocacy Group. 59

Chapter Twelve – Room Service 67

Chapter Thirteen – Journey to Inversion 69

Chapter Fourteen – The Big Pharma Co 73

Chapter Fifteen – The Biotech 83

Chapter Sixteen – The Ethics Committee. 89

Chapter Seventeen – The Patient Recruitment Vendor 95

Chapter Eighteen – The Only Way to Travel 103

Chapter Nineteen – Vegas Villa 105

Chapter Twenty – The Clinical Trials Conference 107

Chapter Twenty-one – The Decentralized Trials Evangelist. . 111

Chapter Twenty-two – The Patient Recruitment Consultant 117

Chapter Twenty-three – The Primary Care Physicians 125

Chapter Twenty-four – The Elevator Pitch Solution. 129

Chapter Twenty-five – The Mentor. 132

Chapter Twenty-six – The Rare Disease Patient 135

Chapter Twenty-seven – The Magic Wand Index 143

Chapter Twenty-eight – Solving the Patient Recruitment

                              Conundrum 151

Chapter Twenty-nine – Let's Work Together. 155

Appendix: Josh's Notes and Mind Maps 157

Preface

There's a famous saying – often attributed to Einstein – that if you have an hour to save the world, you should spend the first 55 minutes defining the problem.

This book is an attempt at those first 55 minutes looking at the problems of recruiting patients for clinical trials.

It's written in the style of a novel so, if you don't wish to wade through my literary pretensions, the summary notes included as an appendix provide an overview of the issues facing each of the main stakeholders in the patient recruitment process.

Chapter One – The Invitation

Josh Black leaned back in the worn leather chair, the flickering glow of the computer screen illuminating the dimly lit room. The soft hum of the microphone lingered in the air as he ended his latest podcast episode. "And that, my friends, concludes today's episode of Humdrum Conundrum. Thanks for joining me as we try to solve some of the world's mysteries, one discussion at a time. Until next week, keep puzzling."

He pressed the stop button and took off his headphones, allowing the silence to settle around him. Podcasting had become the main focus of his activities; a way of solving problems and diving deep into the issues that plagued businesses and cultural phenomena allowing him to offer his unique insights to an eager audience. The word Humdrum in the title was primarily a play on the rhyme with Conundrum but also reflected the commonplace nature of many of the issues he was asked to explore.

As he mused on another successful recording, something else cried out for his attention. More than a flicker of curiosity danced in Josh's eyes as he looked at the envelope lying on the desk. In stark contrast to the digital landscape that dominated his life, this was an old-fashioned piece of paper, sealed in an envelope, bearing his name in elegant handwriting. The return address indicated it came from London, England. Unusual in this age of emails and instant messaging to receive such physical correspondence.

Josh was about to use his fingers to open the envelope then remembered a gift he had received from a grateful client who he had helped to discover the whereabouts of a missing World War Two plane – a letter opener in the shape of a propeller.

He smiled as he carefully ran the side of the blade through the envelope's closure, taking out and unfolding the letter within. Reading the handwritten words – even more unusual in this age of typewritten everything, and in a flamboyant blue script obviously written with an expensive fountain pen – his pulse quickened, a sense of intrigue washing over him.

The letter invited him to a meeting with multimillionaire British businessman, Alexander Wexford, a name that exuded wealth and power. Wexford had recently sold Awex, his contract research organization, making headlines in the life sciences industry with the astronomical figure involved.

The letter provided no specific details about the meeting's purpose, only tantalizing hints of an interesting puzzle for Josh to solve – a challenge apparently related to the most significant problem facing the industry. It stirred something deep within him, a thirst for the unknown and a desire to make a difference. Josh's mind began racing with possibilities, the contents of the letter promising the prospect of uncovering secrets that could shape the future of an entire commercial field.

As he contemplated the mysterious invitation, his gaze shifted to the view outside the window of his home office – a sprawling cityscape that Josh often thought seemed to mirror the twists and turns of the puzzles he tackled on his podcast. The muffled rhythmic sounds of traffic reached his ears, reinforcing within him the idea the world was full of complexities waiting to be unraveled.

Josh had always been drawn to puzzles. Indeed, he had made a career of it with his work for the British and American secret services. Something he occasionally hinted at – but never revealed entirely – on his podcast.

Given what Wexford had written in the letter, something about this potential project seemed to be different from the sort of things Josh usually became involved with. A puzzle that extended beyond the confines of his podcast with an answer that could have real-world consequences. The prospect was unusually exciting, brimming with the promise of doing something with a greater purpose.

With a determined click of the mouse, Josh opened a new browser window on the computer and looked up flights to London. As he did so though, he noticed a postscript in the letter suggesting that if he wished to find out more, he should simply send an email to Wexford's assistant and all travel arrangements would be made on his behalf to set up a meeting between the puzzle solver and the letter writer.

Josh spoke out loud, mimicking the way he might open one of his podcast episodes.

"Well, Alexander Wexford esquire, you've got my attention. Let's see what kind of puzzle you've prepared for me."

And with that, Josh began writing the email that would set him on course to try to solve a mystery that had stumped an entire multi-billion dollar industry for decades.

Chapter Two – Flight into the Unknown

Josh settled into the plush leather seat of the first-class cabin, his fingers tracing the embossed stitching as he embraced the luxury surrounding him. It was a far cry from the budget airline travels he had been familiar with in his youth. Business class had been his usual level for the past few years, but being in a completely separate cabin from the rest of the passengers was a testament to the opulence of Alexander Wexford's invitation. The British businessman had spared no expense, ensuring that Josh's journey to London was as comfortable as possible.

Sipping on a glass of champagne offered by the attentive flight attendant, Josh allowed his mind to wander, contemplating the enigma awaiting him across the Atlantic – back to the country of his birth. The letter had piqued his curiosity, leaving him with more questions than answers. What was the "biggest problem" plaguing the life sciences industry? How did it relate to Alexander Wexford's business empire? And what could Josh do to help to unwrap this puzzle?

The excitement whirred within Josh, mingling with a hint of apprehension. He had solved numerous problems on his podcast, dissecting complex issues and shedding light on the darkest corners of industries and society.

As the airplane soared through the clouds, Josh's thoughts drifted back to the countless hours he had dedicated to his podcast. It had started as a way to share his passion for unraveling mysteries and explaining the various mental models he had put to good use in his career and life. But over time, it had grown into something more – a platform that connected him to a worldwide community hungry for knowledge and eager to engage in thought-provoking discussions.

Humdrum Conundrum had become his medium for impact, his tool for making a difference. Through this podcast, he had helped businesses to overcome hurdles, shed light on societal issues, and sparked conversations that resonated with listeners around the globe. And now, it seemed, Alexander Wexford had recognized the value of his unique perspective, summoning him to London for a challenge that went beyond the confines of his virtual studio.

The possibilities of the opportunity weighed on Josh's mind. If he succeeded in unraveling the puzzle set before him, Wexford had hinted it could effect change on a grand scale, maybe alter the course of an entire industry, and perhaps leave a lasting legacy.

Lost in his contemplations, Josh leaned back, closing his eyes, allowing the soothing thrum of the aircraft to wash over him. Images of his past investigations and discussions flickered through his mind – the faces of business leaders, experts, and listeners who had shared their stories and entrusted him with their secrets.

With every episode, he had learned something new, expanded his knowledge, and honed his analytical skills. Josh wondered if this meeting with Alexander Wexford represented a new chapter – a chapter that would push him further, challenge him to think beyond the confines of his podcast, and venture into uncharted territory, something that, deep down, he realized he had probably been looking for all along.

Opening his eyes, Josh glanced out the window, catching a glimpse of the Atlantic Ocean stretching out beneath the airplane's wings. He wondered if it was symbolic of the vastness of the puzzle he was about to confront, with layers of complexity and depth hidden beneath the surface.

He set about trying to guess what the issue might be. Obviously, he had done some research and come across lots of references on the internet to the problems within clinical trials. Cross-referencing those with what he knew about Alexander Wexford's company, he had come to the conclusion it was probably something to do with recruiting patients that was the issue he was to be asked to look at. But it probably wouldn't do to speculate too much. Better to enjoy the hospitality of the first class cabin including, of course, the selection of wines on offer, and await more information at the appropriate time.

After what seemed like the briefest few moments of sleep, the flight attendant announced their imminent arrival, and Josh awoke with a start, his mind still racing with the ideas that had been forming in his dreams.

The time for speculation and anticipation was over. It was time for action – for puzzle solver extraordinaire Josh Black to step off the plane, enter the world of Alexander Wexford, and confront what he hoped might be the greatest challenge of his career. The stage was set, and the puzzle awaited its solver.

Chapter Three – Hotel Homecoming

Josh stepped out of the black S-class Mercedes that had transported him from the airport to the grand entrance of The Rosemount – one of London's most well-known five star hotels. The imposing structure stood tall, wreathed in elegance and history. Its name was synonymous with luxury, and it was clear that no expense had been spared for his accommodation, courtesy of the forthcoming meeting with Alexander Wexford.

As he approached the reception desk, his luggage having been whisked away at the hotel entrance, Josh couldn't help but be impressed by the opulent surroundings. The lobby was adorned with intricate chandeliers and plush furnishings, solid wood furniture adding to the sense of timeless grandeur. The hotel staff greeted him with warm smiles, seemingly ready to cater to his every need.

"Good evening, Mr. Black," the impeccably dressed receptionist said, her tone tinged with professionalism. "We've been expecting you. Mr. Wexford has made all the necessary arrangements for your stay. Please allow me to check you in."

Josh handed over his identification, his eyes surveying the lobby as he waited. It was a place where royalty and celebrities had graced the halls – sometimes with scandalous results – and now he found himself a part of that exclusive world. A world where solving puzzles and seeking truth appeared to have opened doors he could never have imagined.

The receptionist handed a keycard to an immaculately dressed porter.

"Mr. Black, you'll be staying in one of our largest suites on the top floor. It offers breathtaking views of the city, and comes with all the amenities one would expect from The Rosemount. I hope you'll find it to your liking."

Josh nodded appreciatively, his mind racing with anticipation. As he followed the porter to the lift, he began to run through the possible scenarios that might greet him during the meeting with the benefactor of his current situation.

On arriving at the suite, the porter swung the double doors open, revealing a sanctuary of elegance and comfort. Sunlight flooded into the room, casting a warm glow over the carefully curated furnishings. The room gave off a sense of refinement, offering respite from the outside world and, Josh thought, a perfect setting for contemplation and preparation.

Josh approached the window, drawn to the panoramic view of London's iconic skyline. The city stretched out before him, a tapestry of history, culture, and untold stories. It was a reminder to him of his background, having been born in England and worked there for the early part of his career before moving to America in his early thirties.

Having tipped the porter, wondering as he did so if it was expected in a place such as this, he settled into the comfort of a large cushioned armchair and had more of a look around.

His gaze was drawn to the large wooden writing desk with leather inlay that was situated at right angles to the furthest of the three floor to ceiling windows; the sort Josh could imagine famous writers of old, such as Charles Dickens and Rudyard Kipling, may have been familiar with.

He started to imagine himself setting up his working environment on that desk, maybe even recording a podcast from it – the modern computer and recording equipment a sharp contrast to the old-fashioned workstation it would be placed on.

Content in his ruminations, Josh felt himself giving in to the inevitable jetlag that always followed a trans-Atlantic jaunt, and closed his eyes to get some rest before embarking on the next stage of the adventure.

Chapter Four – Wexford's World of Wealth

The opulent black limousine glided through the streets of London, carrying Josh towards the outskirts of the city. This time Alexander Wexford had sent his own car – a Rolls-Royce Phantom with the registration plate 'AW 1' – and Josh was very much enjoying being cossetted by the hand-finished luxury within.

He watched as the urban landscape slowly transformed into picturesque countryside. The sprawling green fields and quaint villages painting a serene backdrop in stark contrast to the frenetic city he had left behind.

As the 6 meter, 2.5 tonne car made its way majestically through the winding roads, Josh's thoughts swirled with anticipation. The letter from Alexander Wexford had only hinted at the type of puzzle he was about to face, leaving him with a hunger for answers and increasingly intrigued by the enigmatic British business titan.

After just over an hour, the enormous vehicle arrived at its destination – a magnificent mansion nestled amidst meticulously manicured gardens in one of the 'millionaire's row' areas around Ascot. The grandeur of the estate was awe-inspiring, a testament to Alexander Wexford's wealth and taste for the finer things in life.

Josh stepped out of the car, taking in the surroundings. The air carried a sense of tranquility disrupted only by the distant sounds of nature and the soft murmurs of the wind.

As he approached the entrance, the ornate double doors swung open revealing a vast foyer adorned with marble and multiple artworks. Waiting for him at the threshold was a distinguished butler who greeted him and stood to one side.

"Mr. Black, welcome to Wexford Manor," the butler said, his voice resonating with a touch of formality. "Mr. Wexford is expecting you. Please follow me."

Josh followed the butler through the grand corridors of the mansion, their steps echoing on the polished marble floors. The venue seemed to hold a certain aura, a weight of expectancy that matched his own.

After what seemed like several minutes, they arrived at a study – a room brimming with a sense of power and purpose. Bookshelves lined the walls, filled with leather-bound tomes and artifacts from around the world. A large oak desk occupied the center of the room, behind which was the commanding presence of Alexander Wexford himself.

Wexford's inquiring gaze met Josh's as he rose from the chair, extending a hand in greeting. "Josh Black, a pleasure to meet you in person," he said, in an authoritative voice. "Thank you for accepting my invitation. I'm a great fan of your podcast from which I've learned you have a knack for solving puzzles, and I have one that requires your expertise."

Josh shook Wexford's hand firmly, studying the businessman's face for any clues. The anticipation within him grew, eager to delve into the mystery that had brought him here.

"I'm honored to be here, Mr. Wexford," Josh replied, his voice steady. "I thrive on puzzles, and I'm ready to tackle any challenge you present."

Wexford motioned for Josh to take a seat opposite him, their eyes locked in an unspoken understanding. As they settled into the chairs, the room seemed to pulse with an electric energy – an unspoken acknowledgement that something significant was about to unfold.

"Josh, the life sciences industry is at a critical juncture," Wexford began, his tone light but serious. "There's a longstanding problem that has the potential to derail progress, jeopardize lives, and stagnate innovation. It's a puzzle the answer to which has eluded even the brightest minds in the field."

Josh leaned forward, his curiosity piqued. "Tell me more, Mr. Wexford. What is this problem and how is it connected to your business empire?"

A contemplative silence settled between them before Wexford spoke again, his voice now more playful.

"If I have something like the measure of the type of man you are, Mr. Black – which I would be surprised if I didn't – I'm sure you'll already have some idea as to what the issue is."

Josh leaned back again, accepting the implied compliment, and responded with what he had come to believe was likely to be the main issue. "Patient recruitment for clinical trials?"

Wexford smiled and nodded his head.

"Indeed, Mr. Black, indeed. And not just recruitment, also retention – though most often these two elements are bundled together as one. Somewhat ludicrously, patient recruitment is the single biggest issue plaguing the drug development industry. Clinical trials, which are the lifeblood of our efforts to bring new treatments to market, suffer severe delays or even cancellations due to the struggle to enrol and retain patients."

Josh nodded in agreement. The research he had undertaken prior to this meeting had certainly led him in the direction of recruiting patients being the likeliest field that Wexford wanted him to address.

Wexford leaned forward, his eyes intense with determination. "Even my organization, with its track record of success, has fallen victim to this problem. We've witnessed first-hand how patient recruitment and retention can hamper progress, stifling innovation and leaving potentially life-saving treatments stranded in the pipeline."

As Josh listened, his mind raced to connect the dots. Patient recruitment and retention – two sides of the same coin, intricately linked in a battle against time. The lack of participants in clinical trials meant a slower pace of research, increased costs, and limited opportunities to gather vital data.

"The nature of these intertwined challenges is such that they demand innovative solutions," Wexford continued, his voice resolute. "And that's where I believe you, Josh Black, puzzle solver extraordinaire, can make the difference. Your ability to dissect complex issues, uncover insights, and connect with people through your podcast could hold the key to unlocking the problem."

"I understand the significance of this problem, Mr. Wexford," Josh replied, his voice steady. "And I've done a little background research to work out how I might be able to add something useful but, given the fact that even people who are vastly experienced with running clinical trials are unable to come up with a suitable answer, where do we start? What can be done to address the issues that have plagued the industry for so long?"

A faint smile crossed Wexford's face as he nodded appreciatively. "Well, that's for you to determine, Mr Puzzle Solver. But I should think a good place to start would be thinking outside the box, embracing technology, bridging the gap between patients, healthcare providers, and researchers. I should think we might want to investigate a comprehensive approach that combines data analytics, patient engagement, and streamlined processes. And by the way, Josh, I'm committed to providing you with the resources, the connections, and the drive to support you in this endeavor."

The weight of the task ahead settled upon Josh's shoulders, but so did a surge of determination. He was being given an opportunity to make a tangible impact on an industry that held the key to improving countless lives. The challenge presented by patient recruitment and retention resonated with his core values – the pursuit of truth, the search for solutions, and the unwavering commitment to making a difference.

As Josh and Wexford continued their discussion, including the brief mention of a very handsome fee to be handed over for Josh's time, a few ideas began to take shape regarding a puzzle-solving mission that would require collaboration, innovation, and unwavering dedication. The meeting had not been going on for long but the path forward was becoming clearer with each passing moment or, at least, the route to get to the path.

Armed with the resources and support of Alexander Wexford, Josh was determined to unravel the complexities of patient recruitment and retention. It was a journey he thought could test his intellect, resilience, and adaptability, but one that held the potential to transform the landscape of drug development and improve the lives of those individuals in need of a new treatment.

'Bring it on!' Josh found himself thinking, aware that this could be the most difficult task he had faced to date, but nevertheless feeling enthused by the challenge.

Chapter Five – Sarcastic Sidekick

While Josh and Alexander Wexford continued their chat, a new presence entered the room – a man giving off an air of confidence and a hint of nonchalance. With a mischievous smile and a twinkle in his eye, he strode forward, extending his hand towards Josh.

"Josh, meet Max Donovan," Wexford introduced, gesturing towards the man standing beside him. "Max was my right-hand man during my days in gainful employment. He's been through the trenches, knows the industry inside out, and has a wisecrack for every occasion."

Max Donovan grinned and shook Josh's hand with a firm grip. "Nice to meet you, Black," he said, his voice betraying his American roots. "Hope you're ready for some serious eye-rolling moments, because this industry can be a real circus."

Josh could not help but chuckle at how Max was coming across, giving the impression he had seen it all – a cynical, battle-hardened fixer, armed with a repertoire of sarcastic rejoinders. Although his manner would probably be considered grating to some, it was evident that Max's experience and connections in the industry – allied to Alexander Wexford's money and clout – could prove invaluable to Josh's mission.

Wexford stepped forward, placing a reassuring hand on Max's shoulder. "Josh, I believe that with Max's assistance, you'll be able to navigate the complexities of the clinical trials landscape more effectively. Though he also cashed out at the same time as I did, his name still means something, and his connections can open doors that would otherwise remain closed. Consider him your guide and partner in this endeavor."

Max raised an eyebrow, a sly smile playing on his lips. "Yeah, consider me the cynic with connections," he quipped, a hint of mischief in his voice. "But don't worry, Black, I'm sure we'll get along just fine. I've got the inside scoop on the industry's dirty little secrets, and I'm here to make sure you don't step on any landmines."

Josh felt intrigued, and also a slight sense of relief. With Max Donovan by his side, armed with his industry knowledge and biting wit, he should have a valuable ally as he embarked on interviews and investigations. It may be that Max's brash demeanor and strident sarcasm could be an acquired taste, but there was no denying the value he brought to the table.

As the meeting progressed, Max Donovan shared anecdotes, insights, and cautionary tales, punctuating his words with sardonic jabs and witty remarks. He had the valuable ability to cut through the industry jargon and provide a grounded perspective on the challenges that lay ahead.

Josh knew that Max's presence may prove to be both a blessing and a trial. Their personalities might clash, and their approaches to problem-solving may differ but he also recognized the immense value that Max brought.

After a couple of glasses of fine wine had been served by Wexford's butler, attentions focused more directly on the issue at hand.

"So Max," Wexford said, leading them onwards, "why don't you give our esteemed guest an overview of how things work in the world of clinical trials."

Max leaned back in his chair and flexed his fingers together.

"Alright, Black, here's a crash course on what's involved in the clinical trials circus," he said, his tone laced with a mix of irony and obvious expertise. "First, you've got the research sites. These are the hospitals, clinics, and academic institutions where the trials take place. They're responsible for dealing with patients, administering the treatments, and collecting data. Some sites are better than others. Some are efficient, while others can't even manage to change a lightbulb without a committee meeting."

He continued, ticking off another stakeholder on his fingers. "Then there are the CROs – Contract Research Organizations. They're like the middlemen, hired by the trial sponsors – which are usually pharma companies or biotech firms – to manage and operate the trial. They come in various sizes and flavors – global, boutique, country-specific, therapy area specialists. But let me tell you, their efficiency and attention to detail can vary like night and day."

Max paused, savoring a sip of wine before continuing. "Of course, as I mentioned, you've got the trial sponsors themselves – the pharma, medical device companies or biotechs that are footing the bill and pushing their new treatments through the trials. They've got the most to gain or lose financially, so they're the ones calling the shots, designing the trials and setting the timeline.

Then there are Investigator Initiated Studies – that is, trials that are designed and conducted by the same entity. These might be set up by an academic institution, a charity, a hospital, or an individual researcher."

Josh nodded, absorbing the information. The web of stakeholders involved in the clinical trials process was somewhat larger and perhaps more tangled than he had previously realised – each presumably having their own interests and motivations.

"Patient groups can also play a role," Max added, his voice gaining a touch of seriousness. "They may be charities or not, and can advocate for patients' rights, provide support, and help raise awareness about clinical trials. They could be valuable allies in our mission, Black."

Max leaned forward, his eyes narrowing. "And let's not forget the patient recruitment vendors. These guys are like the matchmakers of the clinical trials world. They use various methods – tech solutions, databases, community outreach programs, doctor outreach programs, DCT solutions – which I'll tell you more about as we go along – traditional ads, digital ads, you name it – to find eligible patients and get them to sign up. But their success rates can be hit and miss. It's like a game of trial and error… pun intended."

Max smirked at his own joke before outlining the patient journey within a clinical trial.

"Now, when it comes to patients, they're the volunteers who participate in the trial. They qualify to take part due to their condition and most often their location within traveling distance of a research site. And let me tell you, their journey through a trial is no walk in the park. They start by finding out about the trial – usually either through responding to an advert or by being in a research site's database. Once the patients has learned more about the trial, they can apply to take part.

At this stage, the research site will try to contact them to come in for a screening where they must fit the eligibility criteria for the trial – which means some may not qualify at that point. Also, unfortunately, it's often the case that a large number of the applicants are unable to be contacted by the site, so never get to the screening stage.

If they are able to be contacted, and subsequently qualify for the trial, then comes the informed consent process – when they're given an overview of the risks, benefits, and possible side effects. After that, if they're eligible and they consent to participate, which not everyone does, they're taken on for the trial. Commonly this will involve them being randomized, with double-blind randomization being acknowledged as the 'gold standard' for clinical trials."

Noticing Josh's querying look, Max went on.

"Randomization means some of the participants receive the treatment being tested and some of them receive a placebo – which is made to look the same as the actual treatment, but actually doesn't contain any active ingredient. It's like playing a medical lottery."

He paused, his expression turning slightly somber. "Patients undergo regular visits, possibly intrusive tests, and monitoring as part of the trial, often with little recompense for any time and expenses incurred, and rarely with an actual payment for their efforts. It can be a demanding process – often referred to as the patient burden which, for some people, is very hard considering the potential burden of having their condition in the first place – and not everyone sticks it out until the end, with people who drop out for whatever reason often being categorized as 'lost to follow up'. But those who are retained on the trial provide the data that eventually gets locked away in the database waiting for analysis and the final verdict on the treatment and whether it's suitable for release into the marketplace.

"And, of course, everything is regulated by rules governing the operation of trials – with government agencies and Ethics Committees or Institutional Review Boards overseeing things to make sure everything is above board.

Max leaned back and took another sip of wine, a satisfied look sheathing his face. "So, Black, that's the nutshell version of the clinical trials process. Now, imagine all the challenges, the egos, and the roadblocks we're gonna come across as we dig deeper. It's gonna be one hell of a ride."

Josh nodded, his mind alive with the complexity of the process. The multitude of stakeholders, the intricate patient journey, the different elements that all somehow contributed to making this the challenge it so obviously was.

And yet, as Josh thought through some of the things he had been told, he was still unsure as to why recruiting patients to take part in trials was considered to be so problematic. As with the other puzzles he had explored in his podcast, he knew the best way to get to the heart of the problem was to learn as much as possible about it from as many angles as possible which is exactly what he intended to do – with the help of Max Donovan, and a little support from Alexander Wexford.

Chapter Six – The Journey Begins

The next morning, warm sunlight filtered through the windows of a cozy café as Josh and Max sat across from each other, sipping coffee.

Max drained his latte and leaned across the table. "Alright, Black, here's the plan," he began, his eyes meeting Josh's. "Today, we start with a research site in central London. We'll dive right into the belly of the beast and talk to the folks who are on the front line of patient recruitment and retention."

Josh nodded, his mind focusing on the task at hand. "Sounds like a good starting point," he replied. "What's our approach going to be? With your experience of these type of people, what's the best way for us to gain insights from the representatives there?"

Max flashed a wry smile. "Well, Black, I've got a few tricks up my sleeve," he said, leaning back with a confident air. "First, we need to establish rapport. These folks are used to the clinical trials song and dance, so we need to show them that we're different – that we're genuinely invested in understanding their challenges."

Josh took another sip of his cappuccino. "And once we've established that connection?" he asked, eager to hear more about Max's thoughts on their best strategy.

Max's eyes gleamed mischievously. "Then, my friend, we start asking the kind of questions that will help us – or, more particularly, you – to uncover whatever nuggets that will be useful. We need to discover the hurdles they face, the bottlenecks in the process, the failed approaches they've taken, and the potential solutions they've been toying with. It's all about digging deep, pushing past the superficial answers, and getting to the core of the matter."

Josh smiled at Max's straightforward and no-nonsense approach. It was clear that his experience in the field had honed his ability to cut through the layers of bureaucracy and should be useful in being able to extract the valuable insights they needed.

Max continued, a hint of seriousness creeping into his tone. "We obviously also need to be mindful of their perspectives," he said. "These folks have their own challenges and frustrations. They're dealing with limited resources, tight deadlines, and a constant battle for funding. It's important we try to understand the realities they face on a day-to-day basis."

Josh nodded. He recognized the importance of not just unraveling the problems, but also appreciating the context in which they existed. The stakeholders they would meet were individuals with their own set of pressures and constraints, and understanding those factors would be crucial to finding viable solutions.

As breakfast came to an end, Josh could not help but feel a surge of anticipation. The research site meeting marked the beginning of their journey – an opportunity to gain first-hand perceptions and hopefully lay the groundwork to unlock the mysteries of patient recruitment and retention.

Max stood up, a smile creasing his lips. "Time to hit the ground running, Black," he declared, forcefully. "Let's dive into the clinical trials world and shake things up."

Josh rose from his seat, experiencing the usual mix of wonder and suspense that he felt at the start of every puzzle-solving project. The meeting with the research site representatives would be just the first step in the mission, but Josh thought it could hold the potential to set the tone for the rest of the investigative journey he was excited to be embarking on.

Chapter Seven – The Research Site

The Delphine Medical Institute – an esteemed facility that held a reputation for cutting-edge clinical research – was nestled amidst the exclusive retail outlets and restaurants of Mayfair. An elegant Georgian house, it portrayed an air of tradition mixed with sophistication.

Josh and Max had made their way there via the London Underground – by far the quickest way to get around this teeming city during the day. Arriving at their destination, the entrance to the research site stood tall, its cream-colored exterior contrasting with the vibrant greenery that framed the imposing double doors. Josh wondered what sort of welcome generally awaited visitors to this world of medical innovation and discovery.

Once they had been buzzed into the clinic, a hushed and serene ambiance enveloped them. The reception area, with polished wooden floors and adorned with tasteful artwork, basked in an air of tranquil professionalism. A warm and friendly receptionist greeted them, her voice carrying a calm reassurance.

"Good morning, my name's Sandra. How may I assist you?" she enquired, her eyes glancing from Max to Josh.

Max took the lead, flashing a charming smile. "Good morning. We're here to meet with Dr. Helen Turner."

Sandra nodded and picked up the phone to announce their arrival. After a brief conversation, she hung up and turned back to them.

"Dr. Turner will be with you shortly. Please have a seat," she said, gesturing towards a comfortable seating area.

Josh took a moment to observe their surroundings. The décor was trying hard to balance the grandeur of the original building with the obvious influence of modernity that was implicit with the nature of the building's purpose. The walls were adorned with certificates attesting to the clinic's commitment to excellence in both research and patient care.

He took in the sounds of activity around them – the soft footsteps of medical professionals, the gentle murmur of conversations, and the occasional beep of medical devices that could be heard from along the corridor. Josh made a mental note that the clinic's atmosphere was a subtle blend of the clinical with a sense of warmth and compassion.

He observed the interactions between the reception staff and patients. It was obvious from the reactions of the patients that they felt well cared for and looked after by the Institute's personnel.

After a few moments, a figure emerged from the corridor leading to the examination rooms. Dr. Helen Turner, the esteemed Principal Investigator at the Delphine Medical Institute, approached them with a poised and purposeful stride, her white suit fitting neatly into the environment as she extended a hand in greeting.

"Good morning, gentlemen," Dr. Turner greeted them with a lukewarm smile. "I must apologize for the delay. My schedule is quite packed, but Mr. Wexford's request prompted me to make time to see you. He's been a valuable supporter of our research endeavors."

Josh smiled, grateful for the influence of Alexander Wexford that had secured them this meeting. He at least partially understood the weight of Dr. Turner's responsibilities and appreciated her willingness to spare them some precious moments.

"We appreciate your time, Dr. Turner," Josh responded, "we understand how busy you are, and we're grateful for this opportunity to learn from your expertise."

Dr. Turner nodded, her expression borne from years of professionalism courtesy. "I'm the Principal Investigator for many of the trials we operate here at the Delphine Medical Institute so my primary focus is to keep the trials running, ensuring protocols are adhered to, data analysis, and guaranteeing patient safety. As you can imagine, it keeps me quite occupied."

Max's eyes sparkled. "No doubt, juggling all those responsibilities must be quite a challenge," he remarked. "We're here to delve into the complexities of patient recruitment and retention, two critical areas that have troubled the industry for years. Your insights will no doubt be invaluable to our mission."

Dr. Turner nodded again. "Indeed, patient recruitment and retention pose significant hurdles in clinical trials," she concurred. "In my role, I'm all too aware of the impact these challenges have on the progress of our trials and the potential to make groundbreaking discoveries. If you eventually do manage to solve the problem, I for one would be highly appreciative of your efforts."

Josh leaned forward, his eyes fixed on Dr. Turner. "We believe that by understanding the perspectives of those directly involved in the trials, we can uncover innovative solutions to address these challenges," he said.

Dr. Turner's gaze softened. "I admire your enthusiasm," she replied, "and will do my best to provide you with insights that may shed light on the complexities involved. However, I must warn you that my time is limited, and I am first and foremost committed to our ongoing research."

Josh nodded, understanding the delicate balance Dr. Turner had to maintain, appreciating her willingness to share her expertise despite her busy schedule.

"Mr. Samson," Dr. Turner said, addressing one of the other people in the waiting area. "How nice to see you again. Everything going OK?"

It was evident from Mr. Samson's reply that he was a trial participant and that he also had a lot of respect for Dr. Turner and the way she managed the trials.

"These gentlemen are here on a mission to improve things for patients, among other things," Dr. Turner explained. "Perhaps you'd give them a quick summary of your own experiences as a trial volunteer?"

Mr. Samson told Josh and Max about his experiences in a clinical trial at the Delphine Medical Institute disclosing that, in fairness, not all of them had been good with some irritation being caused by his phone calls not always being answered promptly. Dr. Turner agreed with this and shared Mr. Samson's frustration – pointing out that it wasn't always possible to provide the perfect level of customer service but this was certainly something she would look to improve.

Overall, though, Mr. Samson was very pleased with the way he was treated and had been delighted to be a part of the trial – feeling himself to be the subject of respect and kindness, and viewed as a vital part of the process rather than simply a 'necessary evil' as he had heard other patients say about other trials they had taken part in. He explained how he had been mostly pleased with the level of communication he had had while taking part in the trial, and how he had occasionally been surprised to receive a birthday card or a 'thank you' note; all things that helped to build a stronger relationship that encouraged him to remain a trial participant.

Dr. Turner, Josh and Max all thanked Mr. Samson for his input then turned towards garnering the thoughts of Dr. Turner herself.

"If you'd like to follow me, gentlemen?" Dr. Turner led Josh and Max along an artwork-filled corridor to her office – a room that seemed somewhat at odds with her nature, being strewn with files and boxes.

"Unfortunately, even in a building as large as ours, there just isn't enough room elsewhere to store all the files the regulations insist on," she said, noticing her guests looking around the room. "So I often end up with the overspill in my office as you can see."

She sat behind a functional oak desk, gesturing for Josh and Max to sit opposite and turning the computer screen around for them to see. Without saying anything she clicked on the large number of windows she had open – revealing a multitude of login screens for different software systems. Her frustration was evident as she navigated them through the complexities of accessing the various different programs.

"Welcome to the world of clinical trial software systems," Dr. Turner said with a weary smile. "Each trial sponsor or CRO has their own preferred system and as the Principal Investigator I'm expected to learn and adapt to each one. It's a constant battle to keep up with the ever-changing landscape of trial technologies."

She clicked on the first login screen, entering her credentials to access the system for Trial A. After a brief loading time, the interface appeared displaying a dashboard filled with study protocols, patient data, and reports. Dr. Turner quickly scrolled through the screens demonstrating the functionalities and intricacies of the system.

"This is Trial A's system. It's reasonably user-friendly but, as with all of these, the learning curve is still present," Dr. Turner explained. "Then the real challenge comes when I have to switch to Trial B, Trial C, and Trial D. Each trial has a different system, each with its own set of features, terminology, and navigation. It becomes a juggling act to ensure data accuracy and compliance across all of them."

The process was repeated for Trials B, C and D with Dr. Turner logging in and demonstrating the unique intricacies of each – the varied interfaces, terminologies, and workflows showcasing the challenges she and everyone else in a similar situation faced on a daily basis.

"I would suggest, gentlemen, that these different systems may well be designed to meet the specific needs of trial sponsors or CROs, but they place an immense burden on investigators like me," Dr. Turner said. "Learning and navigating through multiple systems not only slows down the research process but also increases the potential for errors and data inconsistencies."

Josh observed intently, gaining an immediate understanding of the complexities that Dr. Turner encountered on a daily basis. He made a mental note that the lack of standardized systems across trials added unnecessary hurdles and inefficiencies to the already intricate process of conducting clinical research.

"A quick question for you, Dr. Turner," Josh said. "I can see that having to learn and use all these different systems is a hassle but I'm wondering if there's anything specific about this issue that would affect the patient recruitment process?"

Dr. Turner gave a wry grin. "I'm afraid the issue there, Mr. Black, is that we are far less likely to want to use an unfamiliar system – or indeed sign up to manage a trial that uses an unfamiliar system – so our attention is perhaps diverted away from certain specific trials to ones we know we can manage without there being as much of a headache in terms of the technology involved. This means in the long run that we're more likely to close ourselves off from being part of new trials which, in turn, reduces the available catchment area for patients."

Josh nodded in understanding. He could see that forcing sites to use software systems they did not like would lead to less time being spent on those trials and more time given to trials using systems they preferred.

Dr. Turner turned back to the computer. As she closed the final login screen, she looked from Max to Josh announcing "Of course, this is just one of the many challenges we face when trying to manage and administer clinical trials but, if you can help to streamline and standardize these systems, it would be a tremendous leap forward for our industry."

Josh raised a point he'd been considering. "Do you think, Dr. Turner, that the organizations that design the trials in the first place might benefit from including representatives from research sites in the process?"

Dr. Turner smiled, then replied "I do indeed, Mr. Black. Input from those of us 'on the ground' who actually manage and administer trials on a daily basis might go a long way towards reducing some of the unnecessarily timewasting activities forced upon us as well as helping to come up with a more realistic plan for recruiting and retaining patients in the first place."

Then, glancing at the clock on the wall, "before I have to go back to work, I'd like to show you something else."

She opened yet another screen on the computer and described what it was. "This is a list of the potential trial participants who have been sent to us for screening. If you remember the system for Trial A – the one that was at least partially user-friendly – these patients have been referred for that trial."

Josh and Max leaned closer to look at the list of names. Each one was highlighted in red with a cursory set of notes written next to it.

"What you're looking at, gentlemen, is the evidence of a complete waste of time that my staff had to go through in their attempts to bring in even one of these people for screening."

Josh was puzzled. "Where did these names come from?" he asked.

"I think I can probably answer that one," Max piped up. "I assume, Dr. Turner, these are people provided through a central advertising project organized by a CRO?"

Dr. Turner seemed impressed and nodded at him. "Indeed," she replied. "And, as per usual with those, each and every patient referred to us was not suitable to take part in the trial."

"Why?" Josh asked.

"Fundamentally, the advertising campaign undertaken by the firm contracted by the CRO was useless." Dr. Turner replied. "As, I might add, has almost always proven to be the case with those type of campaigns."

Josh looked at her quizzically, prompting Dr. Turner to go on.

"We're always told that central advertising campaigns will provide us with large numbers of pre-screened patients who fit the inclusion/exclusion criteria and are enthusiastic about participating in the trial." She closed down the computer screen. "But the reality is that we receive large numbers of people who either don't fit the criteria at all, or are uninterested or unable to take part."

Max added his own thoughts. "Yes, and I'm afraid the company I used to work for – with Mr Wexford – was often guilty of employing such tactics." He noticed Dr. Turner's facial expression and hurriedly continued "not maliciously, of course. We were often seduced into thinking the solution on offer would genuinely provide pre-screened patients for the trial. Sadly, though, it was rarely the case."

"And if we wish to manage our own advertising projects," Dr. Turner said, "it's quite often the case that sites like this end up having to beg the sponsor for additional funds and go through an interrogation process about how we intend to spend the money and why we think our own input might deliver better results than the central ads the sponsor is already paying for."

Josh made some more mental notes intending to write things up in his usual manner once the thoughts had percolated a little more in his brain.

"Any other problems for you with recruiting patients?" Josh asked.

"Indeed there are," Dr. Turner replied, once again glancing at the clock. "With probably the biggest problem being the lack of unicorns in this vicinity."

Dr. Turner paused, her face implacable, such that Josh could not tell if she was joking or not. "Erm…" he began, before Max interjected once again.

"I believe Dr. Turner is referring to the increasingly strict inclusion/exclusion criteria that accompanies most trials nowadays."

Dr. Turner nodded, continuing what Max had started. "That is indeed it. In the years I've been working in the industry, the criteria that have to be met simply to qualify to take part in a trial have multiplied exponentially. And not in a good way. Hence my reference to unicorns – the one in a million patient who might somehow qualify for a trial. Allow me to demonstrate."

Dr. Turner riffled through a sheaf of papers on the desk and pulled one out and highlighted the multiple criteria that patients must meet in order to be included as a potential participant then pointed out the even larger number of criteria that led to a patient being excluded from being able to take part.

Josh was amazed at the level of detail and could fully understand how this level of qualification would lead to a reduced pool of potential patients for the trial.

"It's quite often the case, somewhat ludicrously," Dr. Turner went on, "that we're attempting to recruit a cohort of super beings to take part in our trial – people with no co-morbidities and no ill effects from the condition they're living with despite the fact we're supposed to be helping to develop new treatments for people who are ill."

Dr. Turner put the inclusion/exclusion document back into the pile of papers, sighing as she took another document from the bottom of the pile.

"And just to compound the problems we face," she went on, "it's a constant struggle to actually get paid what is somewhat erroneously termed 'fair market value'. It certainly appears to those of us in the research site arena that we're very much the bottom rung of the ladder when it comes to respect for our services within the industry. Don't be fooled by the look of these surroundings, gentlemen. It's mostly our private work that pays the bills. Sometimes I think we may as well apply to be a charity for our trials work, given how much it can cost us to actually carry it out."

She showed Josh and Max the document she had retrieved – a contract with a CRO for Trial A – pointing to a figure that appeared to Josh to be a very low fee for each patient the site managed through the trial process.

Dr. Turner nodded at them and checked the time once more.

"And with that, gentlemen, I'm afraid I must curtail our meeting and get back to my day job," she said, ushering them out of the office. "I sincerely hope you can take what I've said here on board and achieve something that the entire industry has been in desperate need of for a very long time" although the look on her face made it clear she was not all that hopeful that they would succeed.

Josh and Max each shook her hand and made their way out of the room. Josh certainly believed he now had more of an understanding of some of the issues involved with the problem he was trying to solve. But he knew there was a lot more to it than these, and there would be more learnings to pick up before he was anywhere near getting close to an answer.

Chapter Eight – Debrief and Download

After the meeting with Dr. Turner, Josh and Max made their way to a bar nestling in one of London's more vibrant neighborhoods – the venue itself seemingly a haven of relaxation amidst the fevered cityscape. The bar emanated a rustic charm with exposed brick walls adorned with vintage posters and dimly lit by softly glowing Victorian-style bulbs.

They settled into a booth tucked away on the far wall affording them a measure of privacy amidst the lively ambiance. Through the large windows, they could catch glimpses of the activity on the city streets outside – the scene a tapestry of colourful characters and alive with energy.

Max leaned back, swirling the drink in his hand as he surveyed their surroundings. "Not a bad spot for a debrief, huh?" he remarked. "The perfect place to unwind and digest all the knowledge imparted so far today."

Josh nodded in agreement, his eyes scanning the room. "Definitely. It's good to have time to reflect on what we've learned so far," he replied. "Dr. Turner provided valuable insights into the complexities of patient recruitment from the perspective of a research site, starting with the challenges of navigating different trial software systems."

Max took a sip of his drink. "Yeah, those software systems are a mess and always have been," he said. "Imagine having to learn a new system for each trial. It's a recipe for inefficiency and errors."

Josh nodded in agreement. "Indeed. It seems clear that the lack of standardization in trial software systems poses significant challenges – not just for Principal Investigators like Dr. Turner but also for the overall integrity and efficiency of the clinical trials process."

As they discussed their findings, the conversation flowed effortlessly, blending analysis and insight with moments of light-hearted banter – the latter provided primarily by Max in his sarcastic way. The bar provided a comforting backdrop to their discussion, a sort of refuge where they could express their thoughts and bounce around some ideas.

They went through the other learnings, such as the lack of quality in central advertising campaign patient referrals, and the difficulties of finding actual human beings who might fit the inclusion/exclusion criteria for most modern trials. And finally, both expressed their amazement at the level of fees that appeared to be on offer to the people on the front line of the industry although Max, of course, had to appreciate the irony of having been involved with this 'race to the bottom' through Alexander Wexford's CRO.

Having reached a consensus on what they had learned, Max leaned forward, his voice carrying a touch of determination. "But you know, Black, despite the challenges we've discovered, I can't help but feel a spark of optimism. There's so much potential for improvement, so many opportunities to revolutionize the way the patient recruitment process is conducted."

Josh smiled. "You're right, Max," he replied. "I'm sure we'll encounter many more hurdles, complexities, and frustrations, but those are the very things that ignite people's passion for improvement. With every challenge comes an opportunity to make a difference. To streamline processes, improve patient experiences, and ultimately transform the landscape of clinical trials."

Their conversation continued – a mix of introspection, analysis, and shared enthusiasm. They dissected the intricacies of the problem, discussed the need for standardized systems, contemplated how to make central campaigns more effective, pondered what would be required for inclusion/exclusion criteria to be opened up to a wider population, and ultimately considered the ways in which their mission could impact the lives of patients and the future of medical research.

As lunchtime drew near, Max explained that he would have to spend the rest of the day on some unconnected business for Alexander Wexford, and that he would be back in touch later that afternoon to give Josh the details of their next meeting.

Josh decided to have lunch where they were then take a look around the area. London was a place he was familiar with from the old days but not somewhere he had visited for a few years so he was keen to soak up some of its atmosphere and find out how this ever-changing city had developed in the intervening period.

Returning to the hotel later that day, he had dinner in the hotel restaurant before retiring to his room to jot down his thoughts so far.

In the tranquil confines of the spacious suite, Josh settled at the ornate wooden desk bathed in the soft glow of a desk lamp. With a notepad and pencil before him, he began to sketch out a mind map – a visual representation of the knowledge he had gained throughout his journey so far.

With a focused gaze, he started with a main node at the center of the page, writing 'Patient Recruitment Stakeholders' in bold letters. From this central point, he extended branches, each representing a facet of the topic that had emerged during the discussions.

One branch represented the stakeholders – research sites, CROs, pharma companies, patients – each playing a distinct role in the clinical trials process. Another mind map outlined the steps in the patient recruitment process he had learned during the initial conversations with Alexander Wexford and Max – from awareness to consent, randomization to treatment, and final visits. Josh used arrows to signify the progression of patients through these stages, highlighting the potential points of friction and the need for a patient-centric approach.

After finishing the mind map based on 'Trial Participation', he tore a new leaf from the pad and jotted down 'Research Sites' in a central bubble then added a branch that captured the complexities of trial software systems – each trial with its own unique system, requiring researchers like Dr. Turner to navigate a labyrinth of interfaces and processes. He then added branches for 'Central Ad Campaigns' and 'Inclusion/Exclusion Criteria' – each with its own set of connected issues plus one for Payments and 'Fair Market Value' – to which he simply added a question mark and underlined the word 'Fair'.

As Josh mapped out the interconnected web of information, the mind map grew, taking shape as a visual representation of the knowledge he had gained thus far.

Once complete, he set about turning the mind map information into written notes – a technique he had come to rely on for his podcast episodes as he found this helped him to both retain the relevant information and clarify his thinking at the same time.

Hours passed in the hotel room with Josh fully engrossed in this task, his mind pulsing with ideas and possibilities. He referred and added continuously to the mind map, adding bullet points and thoughts to his written notes, all the while outlining the complexity of the puzzle he aimed to solve.

Finally, he sat back in the swish leather chair and reviewed what he had done. He checked the time and realized he had better get some sleep – a few hours previously Max had informed him they had an early morning meeting with a representative from Wexford's old CRO firm.

'OK', he thought, tidying the papers and pencil to the side of the desk, 'now the quest has really started.'

Chapter Nine – The CRO

The next morning, Josh and Max met at the appointed hour and embarked on the journey to the office of the Awex Contract Research Organization (CRO) – previously owned by Alexander Wexford, an establishment where Max was well-known and his name still carried weight.

Located near London Bridge, the office occupied a sleek and modern building that rose majestically against the backdrop of the cityscape. Its glass façade gleamed under the morning sun, reflecting the vibrant energy of the surrounding urban landscape.

As Josh and Max approached the building, the sounds of activity grew more pronounced. Professionals in business attire hurried about engrossed in their tasks while murmurs of conversation filled the air. The entrance boasted an impressive lobby with a polished tiled floor and minimalist design accents, portraying an air of efficiency and professionalism.

Max strode confidently through the entrance, his presence commanding respect as he exchanged greetings with familiar faces. The reception area, with its sleek furnishings and contemporary pieces of sculpture, stood as a testament to the CRO's commitment to cutting-edge research and innovation.

Josh followed closely behind, taking in the atmosphere – a blend of hope and purpose that permeated the air. The CRO's solid reputation was one Josh had learned all about, and he felt a sense of excitement mingled with the weight of responsibility, knowing that their mission to uncover solutions for patient recruitment and retention could take a further step within these walls.

As they made their way to a conference room, passing by glass-walled offices and busy workstations, the energy of the place was infectious. The office purred with the collective expertise and dedication of the professionals who strived to advance medical research.

Inside the conference room, floor-to-ceiling windows offered a panoramic view of the city – a feature of Awex's strategic location amid the grandeur of London's skyline. The room itself was well-appointed with a long table and comfortable chairs plus all the associated tech paraphernalia that would enable the room's occupants to host discussions that could one day help to shape the future of clinical trials. This included a 360 degree microphone in the center of the table, multiple plug-in stations, speakers to broadcast the voices of those joining meetings remotely, digital whiteboards for recording thoughts and so forth.

Max's reputation preceded him, and the room's occupants – a middle-aged man, a man in his late twenties, and a middle-aged woman – greeted him with a mixture of respect and curiosity. His wit and expertise had earned him a place of distinction within the industry, and it was clear that his presence brought a certain level of expectation to the meeting.

Josh took a moment to absorb the scene – the dynamic atmosphere, the eager faces, and the air of possibility that filled the room. He was well aware of the challenge ahead so felt a surge of determination, knowing that they were in the right place to uncover further insights and perspectives that would drive their mission forward.

Seated at the table, a distinguished figure caught Josh's attention as he rose to speak. Clad in a well-tailored suit, his salt-and-pepper hair neatly groomed, he radiated an air of confidence and experience. This individual, introduced by Max as Dr. Robert Hastings, was a seasoned executive at the CRO, renowned for his expertise in site feasibility and his dexterity at keeping clinical operations running to budget.

Dr. Hastings began to speak, his voice carrying a rich timbre that Josh knew would command the attention of everyone he worked with. "Gentlemen, allow me to provide some insights into the crucial work of a CRO in the realm of clinical trials. As a CRO, our primary objective is to support and facilitate the execution of clinical trials on behalf of trial sponsors," he explained. "We work closely with them, guiding them through the complex process of bringing a new drug to market."

He went on to describe the critical role of site feasibility in the early stages of trial planning. "Site feasibility is a meticulous process that involves assessing potential research sites to determine their suitability to conduct a particular clinical trial. Factors such as medical infrastructure, access to patient populations, and the availability of experienced investigators all come into play."

Josh observed the others nodding along in agreement as Dr. Hastings emphasized the importance of site selection in ensuring the successful recruitment and retention of patients. "Identifying the right site is crucial for efficient patient recruitment," he stressed. "By partnering with a research site that aligns with the trial's target patient population, we enhance the chances of enrolling eligible participants and hitting our timeline goals."

Josh had already been briefed by Max that Dr. Hastings was an advocate for site feasibility and selection being the main driver of successful patient recruitment and retention. Max had also added, however, that maybe the results did not quite fit with those beliefs.

Dr. Hastings went on, elaborating on some of the additional strategies employed by Awex to improve their patient recruitment activities. "Outside our highly effective site selection methodology… [Max gave Josh a sideways grin at this] … we adopt a range of other strategies, leveraging various tactics and channels to raise awareness and engage potential participants. From collaborating with patient advocacy groups and utilizing physician networks, we leave no stone unturned in our quest to find suitable candidates for the trials of our sponsor clients."

As Dr. Hastings concluded his overview, Josh and Max exchanged glances, impressed by the depth of knowledge and insights he had shared, but at the same time realizing they perhaps were not getting the full story. Josh was starting to further understand the role of a CRO in bridging the gap between trial sponsors, research sites, and patients, while at the same time striving to optimize the recruitment process and enhance the likelihood of successful clinical trials.

As Dr. Hastings sat back down, indicating he had wrapped up his explanation of site feasibility and patient recruitment, Max could not resist injecting some of his trademark wit into the conversation.

"Phew, Doc, you've got us all convinced that site feasibility is the name of the game," Max said. "But tell me, do you ever stumble upon sites that are just plain 'infeasible'? I mean, do you ever come across a research site hidden deep in the Amazon rainforest or on top of Mount Everest?"

There was a smattering of slightly nervous laughter from the other CRO employees. Dr. Hastings responded, no hint of amusement in his expression. "Well, Max, while we haven't quite ventured into the depths of the rainforest or conquered Everest for clinical trials, we do encounter some unique and challenging locations," he replied. "Our job is to find sites that strike the right balance between accessibility and the specific needs of the trial."

Max nodded. "Ah, the elusive search for the Goldilocks of research sites," he jested. "Not too remote, not too crowded, but just right for patient recruitment. I bet you've become quite the expert in spotting those hidden gems."

This time there was slightly more laughter – if anything with a somewhat more nervous edge. Dr. Hastings could tell there was more beneath what Max was saying, but did not want to move from his position.

"Well, Max, it's safe to say that we've become quite skilled at unearthing those 'just right' research sites," Dr. Hastings replied. "But it's an ever-evolving process, as you'll no doubt remember, and we're always striving to find new ways to optimize patient recruitment and retention."

Josh decided to take up the mantle, raising a few concerns based on what he had learned about the ineffectiveness of certain practices.

"Dr. Hastings, I must say that the traditional approach seems to have its flaws," he said. "From what we've gathered so far, it appears that the current method of site selection and feasibility is actually not always perhaps as effective as the industry might like."

Dr. Hastings sat further back in his chair – his colleagues furtively looking anywhere but at him.

Josh continued. "And my own reading of the situation – and forgive me if I've misinterpreted things – is that the site selection and feasibility process almost always has to be heavily augmented through digital advertising and other methods."

Josh could sense Max stifling a grin as he continued. "And I believe from other sources that CROs often have to bring in patient recruitment solution providers to carry out these other processes. Once again, however, it seems that even with all these methods combined, the process can often miss key patient populations and fail to truly engage them. I'm sure you've given a lot of thought to how to address these challenges?"

Dr. Hastings paused before replying. "You're right, Josh," he acknowledged. "The traditional methods do have limitations, and they don't always reach all the potential patients or create a strong connection with them. It's an area that we recognize needs improvement."

He went on to explain the ongoing efforts within the CRO to adapt and explore alternative approaches. "We're actively exploring new channels and strategies to enhance patient engagement and at the same time ensure that we reach a more diverse patient population. We're putting processes in place that will help us to collaborate with patient advocacy groups, Site Management Organizations, research site networks, and other vendors, plus utilize social media platforms effectively, and leverage emerging technologies to bridge the gap and connect with patients in a more meaningful way."

Josh nodded. "It's encouraging to hear there's a recognition of the need for change," he responded. "And as we continue our journey,

Max and I hope to uncover additional solutions that can help to challenge the status quo and maybe create a more patient-centric approach – one that truly addresses the needs and concerns of the patient population in all its inherent diversity."

Dr. Hastings met Josh's gaze. "I believe our shared mission aligns with that goal, Josh," he replied. "It's through the collective efforts of individuals like you and Max, as well as organizations like ours, that we can drive the necessary change and revolutionize the way clinical trials operate."

Everyone nodded and murmured their agreement, in particular when Max added "not forgetting the inspirational support from Alexander Wexford, of course."

Josh changed tack, asking "so, is there anything about your relationship with sponsors and sites that you think could be improved?"

"Oh pretty much everything," Dr. Hastings replied. "The sites don't play ball and always claim to be too busy to respond to our queries. Sponsors don't understand that using people from their procurement department – who are almost duty-bound to try to get the lowest price – rather than those in clinical operations are not necessarily the right people to be negotiating contracts.

And I've always been concerned about the term 'bid defense' which automatically puts the two parties in adversarial mode rather than having them try to come together for the good of the project as a whole.

Then there's the lack of transparency and visibility of the key stats – often obfuscated by the patient recruitment vendors who don't always want us to know what's going on behind the scenes of what they're doing, and quite often don't deliver on their promises."

Max couldn't resist adding a point of his own. "So, Doc, I think it would be unfair of us to give Josh the impression everything is rosy under the hood. In my day there were significant silos between the different departments – as there are in any big company, I guess – such that one didn't really know what the other was doing or have much internal communication with each other."

"Yes, I'm afraid that's still the case," Dr. Hastings replied. "Especially at larger organizations such as ours and a few others. Maybe with the smaller, boutique CROs that doesn't happen. It's something we'd like to get a grip of but unfortunately that just hasn't happened yet."

The conversation continued, covering some of the areas that had already been brought to Josh's attention in the research site meeting with Dr. Turner as well as emphasizing some of the other issues that CROs face when it came to patient recruitment and ending with a commitment from everyone there to do whatever they could to break the current mold and push forward for better results in the future.

Chapter Ten – A Pub Lunch

Seeking some respite after their meeting at Awex, Josh and Max retreated to an inviting pub nearby. As they settled into a corner booth, Max could not resist sharing a few sarcastic remarks about his past experiences. "Ah, the CROs," he remarked, "they always know how to sell themselves, don't they? Promising the moon and stars, but when it comes down to it, their actions often fall short."

Josh chuckled. "Well, Max, you've had your fair share of experiences with them and, might I add, with that one in particular. Care to share a glimpse into the inner workings of the CRO world?"

Max leaned back, sipping his drink before offering his thoughts. "Let me tell you, Black, in my time working with CROs – and though I only ever worked for Awex, I've had lots of dealings with others – I witnessed some impressive performances. They speak of streamlined processes, advanced technologies, and cutting-edge solutions. But behind the curtain, it's not always as seamless as they like to make out."

Josh leaned forward. "So, Max, what can we really expect from a CRO? What do they actually bring to the table?"

Max replied "Black, the reality is that CROs can offer valuable expertise and resources. They have extensive experience in conducting clinical trials, and their knowledge of site feasibility, regulatory requirements, and operational processes can be invaluable. They also provide guidance and support throughout the trial lifecycle.

"But it's important to go beyond the surface-level promises and delve deeper into their track record. I would tell anyone who wants to bring in a CRO for patient recruitment to look for evidence of their ability to effectively recruit and retain patients, and seek proof of their success rates. It's crucial to ensure their actions align with their words."

Josh nodded. "So, essentially, a potential client needs to assess their capabilities and dig deeper to understand their actual performance rather than solely relying on their marketing pitch?"

"Exactly," Max affirmed. "Sometimes that means asking the tough questions, challenging assumptions, and holding them accountable. It's through this level of scrutiny that a sponsor can truly gauge the value a CRO can bring to the table and ensure that they're the right partner for the project."

As the pub hummed with conversation around them creating a backdrop for their dialogue, Josh and Max decided they would stay for lunch to continue their discussions. As they perused the menu, Max took the opportunity to outline their next meeting, scheduled with a patient advocacy group.

"Alright, Black, let me give you the lowdown on our next rendezvous," Max began. "We'll be meeting with a patient advocacy group – a collection of passionate individuals who champion the rights and needs of patients in a particular therapy area. They've got first-hand experience of navigating the clinical trials landscape so this could be both interesting and enlightening."

Josh leaned in, his mind once more focused on the puzzle he had been presented with rather than trying to choose which extra topping to add to his burger. "That sounds promising, Max," he responded. "What sort of thing do you think we can we expect from this meeting? What insights might they offer?"

Max grinned, underlining his own choice of meal with his finger. "Well, my friend, patient advocacy groups are among the unsung heroes of the clinical trials world," he explained. "They offer a unique perspective – shedding light on the challenges patients face, advocating for their rights, and pushing for greater transparency and inclusivity in the research process.

In this meeting, I'm hoping we'll have the opportunity to hear their stories, understand their frustrations, and gain insights into how the current system may fall short in meeting patient needs. They'll give us a glimpse into the reality of being a patient, navigating the complexities of trials, and how patient-centric practices might truly be able to make a difference."

Josh nodded, his eyes flicking back to the menu. "It sounds like a crucial part of the puzzle," he acknowledged. "Their insights should help us to shape our understanding of the patient experience, and ultimately guide our efforts towards maybe creating a more patient-centered approach."

Max grinned again. "Absolutely, Black," he agreed. "Their stories will bring a human perspective to the challenges we're addressing. It's an opportunity for us to listen, learn, and collaborate with those who are at the forefront of fighting for improved patient outcomes."

A waiter arrived to take their orders, prompting Josh to hurriedly choose the Monterey Jack and barbecue sauce, Max opting for fish and chips – both of them belying their origins and choosing a staple dish more widely associated with the other's home country.

The lunchtime ambiance enveloped them, with the rattle of crockery and cutlery and murmurs of conversation providing a backdrop for their own discussion. Max's insights into the upcoming meeting with the patient advocacy group fueled Josh's determination to approach the discussion with empathy, respect, and a genuine desire to understand the issues from the perspective of the patient.

Chapter Eleven – The Patient Advocacy Group

The patient advocacy group was located in a less glamorous part of London than the CRO. Leaving behind the busy streets and polished facades of the city's more prestigious areas, Josh and Max strolled into a neighborhood that projected a different kind of character.

As they navigated the streets, the scenery transformed from grand buildings and upmarket shops to a more down-to-earth landscape. Colorful storefronts and modest residences lined the roads giving the area perhaps a sense of authenticity and community.

Arriving at their destination, Max and Josh spotted the office they were looking for – an unassuming building nestled amidst its surroundings. The exterior bore a humble charm, its painted facade showcasing the organization's name and purpose.

They stepped through the entrance, greeted by a warm and simple atmosphere that contrasted with the more lavish settings they had recently encountered. The interior embraced a homely aesthetic with doctor's office style seating areas, informational posters, and uplifting artwork adorning the walls – a place obviously designed to be a haven of support and understanding.

The reception area, staffed by friendly faces, transmitted a sense of empathy and compassion. As Max and Josh introduced themselves, they were met with welcoming smiles and a genuine appreciation for their visit. The ambiance within the office purred with a quiet strength – a community of individuals united by their shared experiences and commitment to supporting one another.

Led through the office by a staff member, Max and Josh observed the various areas – a gathering room for support groups, counselling spaces, a quiet room, a resource library filled with educational materials. Josh was impressed that this modest but well-organized office served as a hub of empowerment and advocacy, offering solace and resources to patients grappling with a particular type of cancer.

He felt a wave of respect for humanity wash over him as he observed the dedication and resilience of the group's staff and volunteers. It was a stark reminder that the fight against illness was waged not only in prestigious research institutions, but also in the hearts and minds of those directly affected.

As they settled into a meeting room, Max and Josh prepared themselves for the forthcoming discussion. The middle-aged lady who served as the Chair of the patient advocacy group was Elizabeth Bennett whose journey into advocacy began when her daughter, Emily, was diagnosed with breast cancer – a form of cancer that had profoundly impacted their lives.

Elizabeth, a resilient and compassionate woman, had navigated the challenges of her daughter's diagnosis and treatment with determination. As Emily went through the arduous process of surgeries, chemotherapy, and radiation, Elizabeth faced the daunting task of providing unwavering support on her own.

Recognizing the need for connection, guidance, and understanding, Elizabeth sought solace in some of the patient advocacy groups that specialized in breast cancer support. Through these groups, she found a lifeline – a community of individuals who understood the struggles, fears, and triumphs that she and Emily were facing.

Empowered by the support she received, Elizabeth became deeply involved in the patient advocacy scene, offering her experiences, insights, and empathetic nature to others navigating similar journeys. Her commitment to the cause and her unwavering dedication to the patients and families eventually led her to assume the role of this particular organization's Chair.

Seated around the table, Elizabeth, Max, and Josh began to engage in a heartfelt conversation. Elizabeth, as the Chair, passionately described the purpose and principles that guided the organization.

"Our group is founded on the belief that patients deserve more than just medical treatment," Elizabeth began. "We aim to provide a supportive community, resources, and a voice for those affected by breast cancer. One of our core principles is to prioritize the well-being and best interests of patients. We advocate for access to quality care, improved treatments, and greater transparency in the medical field.

Sponsors, CROs, and patient recruitment firms often approach us, seeking access to our patient database but we have staunchly resisted the idea of selling those details because we believe that many of these organizations are primarily motivated by financial gain rather than a genuine commitment to helping patients."

Josh nodded. "So, you're wary of the intentions of these organizations and how they may exploit the patient data for profit, rather than truly advancing patient care?" he asked.

"Exactly, Josh," Elizabeth affirmed. "We've witnessed many instances when patient data is treated as a commodity rather than a means to improve treatments and quality of life which is why we prioritize the protection of our members' privacy and the ethical use of their information."

Josh leaned forward. "Given your stance, would it be possible for you to navigate collaboration with any of these organizations while ensuring that patients' interests are safeguarded?" he enquired.

Elizabeth smiled, thinking of various instances when they had done just that. "We believe in fostering true partnerships with organizations that share our values and are genuinely committed to patient well-being," she explained. "We seek collaborations where our members' voices are heard, where the focus is on improving treatments, enhancing patient experiences, and driving meaningful change.

We look for organizations that are open about their intentions, uphold rigorous ethical standards, and prioritize patient-centered practices. Our goal when it comes to collaboration is to work hand-in-hand with those who genuinely want to make a positive impact and improve outcomes for patients."

Max and Josh absorbed Elizabeth's insights, recognizing the patient advocacy group's unwavering commitment to safeguarding patients' interests and the need for responsible collaboration within the clinical trials landscape. One of the things Josh picked up on as Elizabeth continued her explanation was how patient advocacy groups would potentially be willing to help to educate their community about available trials by partnering with sponsor organizations to deliver webinars and other types of communication.

As the conversation unfolded, Max introduced a little of his signature light-hearted touch into the discussion. "Well, Elizabeth," he said, "it's refreshing to see a patient advocacy group that doesn't simply roll over and play dead when clinical trial organizations come knocking. Kudos to you for standing your ground."

Elizabeth chuckled. "Thank you, Max," she replied. "As you'll no doubt realise, it's quite the norm for patient groups to be hands-off when it comes to approaches from outside. To take things a little further than others, though we've learned to be vigilant and discerning. After all, the road to meaningful change is often paved with skepticism and a healthy dose of sarcasm."

Josh chimed in. "So I'm assuming, Elizabeth, that your thoughts on involving patients at every stage of the clinical trials process are that it's a desirable thing?"

Elizabeth's eyes sparkled with enthusiasm. "Josh, involving patients at every stage is not only desirable, it's also essential. Patients bring a unique perspective and lived experiences that can shape trial design, inform consent processes, and even influence how treatments are marketed which brings benefits to the study – reducing costs, better retention rates, and providing better health outcomes for patients.

By actively engaging patients, we can ensure that their voices are heard, their needs are addressed, and their experiences are valued throughout the entire clinical trials journey. Not only that, having patients embedded in the research process helps with empathy and encourages people to stay on the trial as it can appear as though trial participants are 'letting their own tribe down' if they see there's someone with the same condition involved in conducting the research. And, obviously, trial volunteers are more likely to be honest and open with a fellow patient rather than someone they might view as simply a researcher."

Max decided it was time for another quip. "I suppose we can't rely solely on the wisdom of white-coated scientists and marketing gurus, can we? After all, patients might have a thing or two to say about what actually matters to them."

Josh posed a couple of follow-up questions. "Elizabeth, how do you think we might go about bridging this obvious gap between patient advocacy groups and the organizations looking to recruit patients for trials? How can we foster a more collaborative approach that truly incorporates patient perspectives and build trust between the two communities of patients and researchers?"

Elizabeth's eyes gleamed with passion as she replied, "Josh, it starts with building relationships and breaking down barriers. We need open lines of communication, transparency, and a willingness – and I agree that this needs to be on both sides – to truly listen and learn from one another. By establishing trust and nurturing partnerships, we can create a space where patient advocacy groups and sponsors, CROs, etc. can work together toward the common goal of improving patient outcomes."

Max asked a question that had occurred to him while listening to Elizabeth. "I'm wondering, Elizabeth, if your group may be something of an outlier in terms of having someone such as yourself at its helm? What I'm thinking is that there are probably many groups who don't have such an articulate and well-connected advocate as you, and whether that affects the level of partnering that is open to them?"

"That's a very good point, Max," Elizabeth replied. "And leads to something that I think would certainly improve the situation for everyone – which is that the CROs themselves should take more action when it comes to engaging with patient groups. If better

connections were made earlier in the process, better results would surely be forthcoming.

"And furthermore, in situations where we do have good engagement from all the relevant stakeholders, it's vitally important that there are effective feedback loops, so that everyone can be kept well-informed throughout the process and help to refine things for the better as we move along."

Her words resonated with Josh, reinforcing the thoughts he had already started having about the importance of collaboration and the need for patients – as well as other stakeholders – to be active participants in shaping the research and development process.

It was clear that Elizabeth believed that involving patients at every stage would lead to more patient-centric clinical trials, ultimately resulting in better outcomes and improved treatments. And it certainly seemed to Josh that she might just be on to something.

Chapter Twelve – Room Service

After Josh and Max had bid farewell to Elizabeth and the patient advocacy group, expressing their gratitude for the enlightening conversation, Josh proposed reconvening later to delve deeper into their insights. However, Max had an unexpected plan up his sleeve.

"Actually, Josh, I've managed to snag tickets for the hottest show in town – 'Rock the Blues'," he exclaimed. "It's a musical extravaganza, showcasing the best blues rock songs of the sixties and seventies. I'm a huge fan so couldn't pass up the chance to experience it!"

Josh smiled. "That sounds incredible, Max. Enjoy the show, I'll catch up with you later," he replied, a tinge of envy in his voice.

They parted ways, Max heading off to immerse himself in the theatrical spectacle while Josh made his way back to the hotel room. Opening the door, he was greeted by the familiar comfort of the temporary abode – a sanctuary of opulence where his thoughts could flow freely.

Settling into the room, Josh cleared a space on the desk and retrieved a fresh sheet of paper. With a mind full of ideas and insights from the day's encounters, he began to sketch out another mind map to represent the knowledge he had gained.

As Josh meticulously connected concepts and ideas, he reflected on the conversations, insights, and perspectives that had shaped his understanding of the clinical trials landscape so far. Patient recruitment, site feasibility, the role of advocacy groups, and the need for patient involvement all found their place on the paper, building into a tapestry of interconnected thoughts and possibilities.

Midway through his task, Josh's hunger made itself known, reminding him of the need to refuel. He decided to order a room service meal, selecting a luxurious dish that would satisfy both his palate and his desire for a moment of indulgence.

Awaiting the meal's arrival, Josh continued mind mapping, allowing the flow of his thoughts to guide his pen. The solitude of the hotel room provided the ideal backdrop for introspection, enabling him to dive deeper into the complexities of the industry and explore the thoughts that occurred based on the challenges faced.

Later, with his plate clean and the evening wearing on, Josh found solace in the quietness of the room knowing that Max was experiencing a very different kind of environment at the theatre. He knew they would reconvene the next day – Max having informed him they were due to visit a big pharmaceutical company – and was looking forward to taking the next steps in the journey.

Chapter Thirteen – Journey to Inversion

As the train glided through the English countryside, Josh and Max settled into the first-class carriage, ready for the next leg of the journey – a global pharmaceutical company based in Oxford. The plush surroundings provided an air of comfort and privacy, allowing them to engage in a conversation that blended their past experiences with their current mission.

Max started the discussion. "So you obviously know a bit about my background, Black, but all I really know about you is from your podcast. Well, that and the file that Alexander provided me with," he winked.

Josh leaned back, his gaze fixed on the passing landscape outside the window. "Well, Max, my background as a cryptographer for GCHQ and a troubleshooter for an international management consultancy is out there for all to see. Maybe I'll tell you some stories about it one day. But perhaps not just yet."

Max smiled, realizing he was not going to get any more from Josh until they knew each other better.

Josh continued. "One of the things that varied background has taught me, of course, is the power of different mental models when approaching problems."

Max looked at him with the expression of someone wanting to know more.

Josh went on. "One technique that's often yielded surprising results is called 'inversion' which is when you deliberately set out to develop a system or approach that would be the worst possible for what you're trying to achieve," he explained.

Max chuckled. "Inversion, huh? Doing things the worst possible way sounds pretty much like the way most patient recruitment projects are currently set up. Whoever develops them already seems to have perfected the art of doing everything wrong."

Josh gave a broad smile. "You might have a point there, Max," he agreed. "It seems that most current approaches to patient recruitment and retention are plagued with inefficiencies and missed opportunities."

He launched into an anecdote, recounting his experience helping a struggling car company overcome manufacturing inefficiencies. "I applied the technique of inversion to that project, imagining the worst possible manufacturing system and working backwards from there. By doing so, we uncovered the root causes of their problems and developed innovative solutions that transformed their production process."

Max leaned forward. "So you're thinking we could beneficially use inversion to tackle the challenges of patient recruitment and retention?" he asked.

Josh nodded. "Exactly, Max. By imagining the worst possible system for patient recruitment, we can identify the pitfalls, the bottlenecks, and the shortcomings that currently exist. And from there, we can systematically address those issues and design a – possibly patient-centric – approach that helps to improve the entire process."

"Interesting stuff, Black. I think you might be onto something there," Max affirmed. "By embracing inversion and challenging the status quo, we can turn the current inefficiencies on their head and pave the way for a successful approach."

The train skimmed along, carrying Josh and Max closer to their destination. They shared a moment of reflection, knowing this possible strategy – borne from the technique of inversion – could hold the potential to reshape the landscape of patient recruitment and retention.

Chapter Fourteen – The Big Pharma Co

Stepping out of the taxi, Josh and Max found themselves standing in front of the grand entrance of the pharmaceutical company's head office. The sleek glass facade and modern architecture displayed an air of success, with perhaps a whiff of the type of profits that awaited those firms that could successfully navigate the clinical trials landscape.

As they entered the building, the swish reception area enveloped them with prestige and professionalism. Immaculately dressed staff hurried about, attending to the needs of visitors – the sum of the parts creating an atmosphere that conveyed the significance of the work being conducted within those walls.

A welcome desk assistant approached, a familiar face to Max. With a mischievous glint in his eye, Max exchanged banter with him, highlighting their shared history.

"No need to point out the enormous list of blockbuster drugs on the wall, Hugo," Max said. "I'm sure Mr. Black here has already clocked it."

Sure enough, taking pride of place in the lobby was a sculpted bronze wall with 33 plaques on it – each of which spelt out the name and history of a best-selling drug that had been developed by this organization.

Hugo was about to point out some other features of the wall when Max stepped in. "And, of course, we're all very impressed with your mission statement to put patients, not profits, at the heart of everything you do, at the same time creating exceptional value for healthcare professionals the world over."

Despite the friendly banter with Hugo, Max made it clear that he would only proceed with the meeting if someone from Research & Development and/or Clinical Operations was present – underlining his determination to engage with key decision-makers.

Complying with Max's request, Hugo arranged for the meeting to include Dr. Rebecca Chambers, the Executive Vice President of Clinical Operations, Global – a respected figure within the company who had worked her way up through the ranks. Accomplished and knowledgeable, she bore the weight of her position with authority and a deep understanding of the intricacies of the clinical trials landscape.

Hugo and Dr. Chambers guided Josh and Max through the impressive office space, a hive of activity where researchers, data analysts, and clinicians collaborated to bring potentially life-saving treatments to the world. All the while, Max was whistling a familiar tune – one that Josh knew but could not place – presumably one he had heard the previous evening at the theatre.

Arriving at the meeting room, a space adorned with modern furnishings in the corporate colors, Josh and Max prepared themselves for the discussion. Dr. Chambers, with her keen intellect and commanding presence, embodied the company's commitment to innovation and excellence.

As the meeting commenced, Josh seized the opportunity to dive straight into the heart of the matter. Fixing his gaze on Dr. Chambers, he posed his first challenge.

"Dr. Chambers, I've always wondered why clinical trial sponsors don't involve patients in the design process. After all, they're the ones who'll be directly affected by the treatments being developed," he enquired.

Dr. Chambers, a seasoned professional with a deep understanding of the industry, acknowledged the importance of patient involvement. "You raise a valid point, Josh," she replied. "While patient involvement in trial design is crucial, there are various factors that contribute to the historical lack of such involvement.

Clinical trial design requires careful consideration of scientific, regulatory, and logistical aspects. In the past, the focus was primarily on meeting strict criteria set by regulatory bodies and ensuring scientific rigor. However, we now recognize the need to shift toward more patient-centric trial design that incorporates the unique perspectives and needs of patients."

Josh nodded. "That's encouraging to hear," he acknowledged. "Patient involvement can surely lead to more relevant trial designs, ultimately increasing the chances of successful outcomes and better patient experiences."

Eager to find out more, Josh raised another challenge. "Another issue we've noticed is the eligibility criteria for trials," he said. "They often appear to be searching for 'unicorn patients' who fit very strict criteria, making recruitment incredibly challenging. Why is this the case, and what can be done to address it?"

"The inclusion/exclusion criteria in trials serve multiple purposes," Dr. Chambers explained. "They're intended to ensure patient safety, reduce potential confounding factors, and maintain the integrity of the study. However, we do, of course, recognize that overly restrictive criteria can limit patient enrolment and result in slower recruitment.

We're actively working to strike a balance between maintaining scientific rigor and inclusivity. By engaging with patient advocacy groups, listening to patient perspectives, bringing representatives from research sites on board, and leveraging advancements in technology, we aim to develop more realistic and flexible criteria that reflect real-world patient populations."

"That's a positive step forward," Josh remarked. "By widening the pool of eligible patients, you can enhance recruitment rates and ensure that trial results are more applicable to the broader patient population but it still doesn't really address the fact that eligibility criteria are often so strict that it's almost impossible to find anyone who fits them."

Max settled back a little further in his chair, appreciating the way Josh was trying to get to the crux of the matter.

"OK, you've raised an important point, Josh," Dr. Chambers responded. "Essentially, the criteria in clinical trials are carefully crafted to meet regulatory requirements and ensure that the treatment under investigation has the best chance of being approved in the necessarily controlled environment not to mention the additional complexities of then having treatments that are approved for use by patients becoming available through the processes involved in market access for pricing and reimbursement issues.

By setting specific criteria, trials can demonstrate the treatment's efficacy and safety in a controlled environment which provides the necessary evidence to gain regulatory approval, thus allowing patients to access the treatment.

However, it's important to note that once a treatment enters the market, ongoing studies are conducted to evaluate its effectiveness and safety in the real-world setting. This stage provides an opportunity to assess how the treatment performs in a wider population, including those who may not have met the strict criteria of the initial trials."

Josh absorbed this information, thinking through the delicate balance between regulatory requirements and real-world applicability. "So, having more inclusive criteria from the start – i.e., that would allow for a broader cross-section of people to participate in the trial – could actually restrict the number of treatments that are ever approved?" he asked.

Dr. Chambers nodded. "Indeed, broadening the criteria from the outset would require a significant shift in the regulatory requirements – and possibly even the business model - of pharmaceutical companies," she confirmed. "The investment of billions of dollars in each new treatment necessitates a carefully designed process to maximize the chances of long-term success and recoup the substantial research and development costs. The cost involved in having a potential treatment fail its trial can be quite enormous, I'm afraid."

Max interjected. "Sounds like the classic catch-22 situation," he said. "To get treatments to market and recoup the investment in R&D, we need narrow criteria, but that limits the number of potential patients who can take part in the trial. It's a tough knot to untangle."

Dr. Chambers smiled. "You've captured the essence of the challenge, Max," she replied. "The delicate balance lies in finding ways to improve trial design and recruitment while ensuring that treatments can move through the regulatory process effectively. And, of course, the Investigator Initiated Trials can help with expanding the patient population for a particular treatment beyond the original eligibility criteria by trialing them for a different indication from that which they've already been approved for."

Max went on to suggest he had often come across trial protocols where substantial elements were simply copied and pasted from earlier trials. The downside of this, he remarked, could be unnecessary eligibility criteria being incorporated in the new trial, which would limit the potential audience.

As the meeting continued, the participants delved further into the intricacies of the regulations and business model, exploring potential opportunities to bridge the gap between having to have rigorous clinical trials and being useful to people in the real-world with all their different co-morbidities and health issues. The candid discussion highlighted the complexity of the issue and underscored the need for innovative solutions that could hopefully drive transformative change within the industry.

They also touched on some issues that had been raised by the CRO – namely the sites or vendors not providing visibility of what was happening, plus the overestimation of their capacity to recruit patients.

Dr. Chambers also raised the issue that they often faced an 'A team, B team' approach when it came to the bid defense process – where the CROs put forward their best people to win the contract then switched over to lower-ranking personnel to manage the project once it was underway. She suggested a more strategic partnership approach between sponsors and CROs would help to eliminate this issue.

"Another thing we often have to deal with," Dr. Chambers went on, "is the global nature of some of the trials we run. This obviously brings its own challenges relating to cultural differences, translations, different inclusion/exclusion criteria, different practices in different territories, the logistics of getting the treatments delivered etc."

After a while, Max raised something he had frequently come across in his career – something he had already mentioned in the meeting with the CRO. "Rebecca, you and I both know that the world of big pharma is perhaps not as smooth-running as it might look from the outside."

Dr. Chambers tilted her head, encouraging him to go on with his point.

"One of the biggest problems I came up against – and I can hardly believe it will have changed – is the silos within the big firms that prevent one department from talking to another, never mind having any clue what they might be doing."

Dr. Chambers nodded almost imperceptibly, moving slightly further back in her chair. "Nope, you're right. It's still a big problem, the main result of which in terms of patient recruitment, I guess, is the clinical team not talking to procurement before the clinical operations vendors are brought in with procurement, of course, wanting to get everything done as quickly as possible without paying over what they define as fair market value while the clinical team wants to get things done as effectively as possible."

"And I have to say it's always puzzled me," Max said, "why your sales teams aren't tasked with informing doctors about clinical trials as well as trying to peddle the latest drugs. With awareness of trials being one of the main roadblocks that prevents healthcare professionals introducing the concept to their patients, surely this could be a worthwhile thing to do?"

Dr. Chambers seemed a little surprised by this. "Well, Max," she replied, "it's interesting you say that. There are compliance issues for sales, of course, and maybe our Medical Science Liaisons, MSLs, are the right people. Something I'll raise at our next internal meeting to see if there's any appetite for it."

Max smiled as Josh made another mental note to explore these aspects of large pharma operations, and how they might benefit from better internal communication. At the same time, he noted down the factors that Dr. Chambers raised such as CROs, research sites, and vendors often wildly overestimating the number of patients they would be able to recruit for a specific trial and also that it was often difficult to get any real sense of how things were going as the updates and reports provided were not always of a high standard.

"And of course," Max added, "it's never fully been explained to me how you can keep a list of preferred suppliers that has dozens of companies on it. How much preference are you really giving one organization over another in that situation?"

Moving on, Josh raised another critical concern. "Dr. Chambers, while diversity is often discussed, the reality is that the majority of clinical trial participants are still predominantly white males. And it's not just about ethnicity; it extends to economic diversity, sexuality, and even – somewhat ludicrously – the underrepresentation of women. How does your approach address this pressing issue?"

Dr. Chambers nodded in agreement. "You're absolutely right, Josh. Diversity is a crucial aspect of clinical trials, and we recognize the need to address this longstanding disparity."

Max snorted and made an observation. "I must say, Rebecca, that diversity, equity and inclusion was being talked about even while I was coming up through the ranks of the industry. Certainly seemed to be little more than a checkbox exercise then, of course."

"I can't disagree, Max," Dr. Chambers replied, "but at the same time I feel it's better to move on with a sense of purpose for the future rather than dwell on what might have been the failings of the past.

At this company, we've developed robust guidelines to ensure diversity in clinical trials that go beyond the recommendations provided by regulatory bodies such as the FDA in the DEPICT act and elsewhere. We actively strive to recruit a more representative participant population through some of the methods mentioned before – such as engaging with diverse communities, leveraging patient advocacy groups, and implementing targeted outreach programs.

And by developing relationships with organizations and communities that reflect a wide range of backgrounds and identities, we aim to increase diversity and ensure equitable access to clinical trials."

"It's encouraging to hear that your company has taken a proactive approach," Josh remarked. "And by implementing stronger guidelines, I agree you have the potential to create a more inclusive landscape that better represents the diverse patient population."

The conversation continued, serving as a reminder of the necessity to consider all dimensions of diversity, including ethnicity, gender, socioeconomic status, and sexual orientation, in order to foster more comprehensive and inclusive clinical trials – something Dr. Turner underlined was now far more prevalent in people's thinking.

Remembering their earlier discussion with Dr. Turner, Josh underlined the point that, as well as patient involvement, having research site involvement from the outset would appear to make sense – with the people 'on the ground' presumably being well-placed to offer assistance regarding ensuring the success of a trial's recruitment and retention strategies.

As the meeting progressed, Josh found himself entranced by the continuing sparky dialogue between Max and Dr. Chambers – an obvious indication that their paths had crossed several times before. But more than this, he knew he was beginning to understand things a lot more clearly, and would be in a much better position to try to solve the puzzle as a result of this visit.

He also wondered what differences he might find in approaches between this huge global enterprise and their next destination – a small biotech firm with, as yet, no product on the market.

Chapter Fifteen – The Biotech

As they got out of the taxi at the science park – home to the emerging biotech firm they were about to meet with – Max turned to Josh with a teasing grin. "Well, Black, here's to the upstarts who are still waiting to make their grand entrance," he remarked. "Let's see what these biotech whizz-kids have up their sleeves."

"Indeed, Max," Josh replied. "Be interesting to witness the cutting-edge developments and fresh perspectives that biotech companies might bring to the table."

Once inside the building, having informed the receptionist who they were there to see, Josh and Max were met by a charismatic individual with neatly styled dark brown hair – his eyes sparkling with a mix of intellect and enthusiasm.

"Hello, gentlemen!" the owner of the biotech firm said, extending a hand in greeting. "I'm Dr. Dan Kumar, founder and CEO of this innovative venture."

He held out his hand for them to shake. "And do please call me Dan," he went on.

"I thought we'd conduct our business in more convivial surroundings," he suggested, leading them to a nearby bar situated in amongst the scientific buildings.

"Thirsty work, saving the world, you know," Dan grinned, settling them into a booth before enlightening them with his thoughts.

"Josh, Max, one of the key differences between big pharma and biotech firms lies in funding and available resources," Dan began. "Big pharma companies often have more significant financial resources at their disposal enabling them to invest in a wide range of research and development initiatives."

He gestured for one of the waiters to come to take their order then continued. "On the other hand, biotech firms – especially those in their early stages – rely heavily on securing funding and support from investors and backers. Once we get past the proof of concept and preclinical stage, some of this funding is contingent upon demonstrating promising results at the initial stages of clinical trials, often serving as a gateway to further financial backing and resources.

The success of passing early stage trials becomes crucial for biotech firms as it opens the door to the sufficient funding required to navigate through subsequent stages which can pose challenges and complexities in the patient recruitment process as the availability of funding is closely tied to trial outcomes."

Josh and Max nodded in understanding, recognizing the high stakes involved for these emerging biotech firms. The precarious journey of progressing through trials, securing funding, and effectively recruiting patients became clearer as Dan shared his insights.

"It's a delicate balancing act," Dan went on. "The need to demonstrate the efficacy and safety of potential treatments in order to secure funding can create pressures that affect patient recruitment and the overall pace of progress.

But while the funding landscape for biotech firms can introduce complexities, it also drives a sense of urgency and innovation. It pushes us to seek creative solutions and forge strategic collaborations to overcome these hurdles and advance our potential treatments."

They paused for a moment while the waiter poured the wine Dan had ordered before Josh asked a question.

"One thing I'm assuming, Dan," he said, "is that, as a smaller biotech, you're not likely to be tied in to a long-term contract with one of the large CRO firms. Of the type this fella used to work for."

He tilted his head toward Max who grinned and raised his glass in acknowledgement.

Dan also grinned and nodded. "That's an interesting one, Josh. Many people who work in biotechs have come from big pharma and simply bring their CRO relationship with them. Whereas in my opinion, the smaller and newer biotech firms can have more flexibility in their choice of clinical outsourcing partners. Unlike big pharma companies that may have long-standing relationships with default and preferred vendors, smaller biotech firms like ours have the opportunity to explore various options and find partners to align with our own unique needs and objectives.

In fact, I'm aware of several instances where smaller firms have bypassed the use of a traditional CRO altogether when it comes to patient recruitment. Instead, they've opted to work directly with patient recruitment specialists, leveraging their expertise in reaching and engaging with the target patient population."

Each of them took a sip of wine, digesting the information being imparted.

"Additionally, there are smaller, boutique CROs that offer a more agile and flexible service that can cater to the unique needs of emerging biotech firms," Dan added. "These nimble organizations can often provide a more tailored and responsive approach, fostering a collaborative partnership between the biotech firm and the clinical operations team which can be very handy for a firm the size of ours.

As you might imagine, I have to wear several hats – often two or three at the same time – which has the benefit of enabling me to make quick decisions but sadly can prevent me from being able to spend much time learning about the sort of solutions that are being developed to help us on our way."

Their discussions continued – helping to shed light on the ever-evolving landscape of clinical operations in the biotech sector. Josh made a mental note that the ability of smaller firms to forge innovative partnerships and explore alternative pathways demonstrated their agility and adaptability, enabling them to navigate the complexities of patient recruitment and leverage specialized expertise.

At the same time, it appeared that this collaborative approach was something worth exploring. Something he would be sure to muse on further when jotting down his thoughts later that evening.

Dan bid them farewell and returned to his office, leaving Josh and Max to plan out their next meeting with a representative from an Ethics Committee (EC), also known as an Institutional Review Board (IRB).

"You know, Black, no matter what patient recruitment firms,

CROs, or sponsors do, they still have to go through the scrutiny and approval process of IRBs or ECs," Max remarked. "It's at the IRB level where the ethical considerations of the trial are assessed, and the protection of participants is evaluated."

Josh nodded, acknowledging the significance of their forthcoming meeting. "Absolutely, Max. It'll be interesting to see what the EC says about ensuring that clinical trials uphold the highest ethical standards and prioritize the safety and well-being of participants," he responded.

They continued their conversation, exploring the intricacies of the IRB approval process and the impact it had on patient recruitment. They discussed the need for transparency, thorough documentation, and adherence to rigorous ethical guidelines to gain the trust and approval of the IRBs or ECs.

Max, ever the skeptic, chimed in with a sarcastic remark. "Well, let's hope they don't slow us down too much with their endless questions and bureaucracy," he said.

Chapter Sixteen – The Ethics Committee

The next morning, Max arrived in Josh's hotel lobby, laptop in hand, ready for the upcoming video calls. They made their way to a designated conference room within the hotel where they prepared for their virtual meeting with a representative from an Ethics Committee.

Setting up the laptop, Max ensured a stable internet connection, and they joined the call, eagerly awaiting insights from the representative who would shed light on the inner workings of this most mysterious of entities.

As the video call commenced, Dr. Emma Mitchell, with her warm smile and aura of approachability, instantly put Josh and Max at ease. She possessed a wealth of experience and a deep understanding of the role that ECs played in the clinical trials landscape.

Dr. Mitchell began by providing an overview of the EC's responsibilities and processes. She emphasized the pivotal role of ECs in safeguarding the rights, safety, and welfare of trial participants. Her voice carried a sense of authority accompanied by a genuine compassion and commitment to ethical considerations.

She delved into the intricacies of an EC's review process, highlighting the importance of evaluating the scientific merit, ethical implications, and potential risks and benefits of proposed trials. Dr. Mitchell stressed the need for transparency, informed consent, and adherence to rigorous ethical guidelines throughout the entire trial process.

With expertise and eloquence, Dr. Mitchell detailed the meticulous nature of the EC's review process, their thorough evaluation of trial protocols, patient information sheets, and informed consent documents. She explained how the committee was composed of diverse professionals, including researchers, clinicians, ethicists, and patient representatives, each bringing their unique perspectives to the table.

Dr. Mitchell emphasized the commitment of ECs to ensuring that trials were conducted with the utmost integrity, maintaining a balance between scientific progress and the ethical considerations that underpin the well-being of trial participants. She underlined their dedication to promoting patient-centric approaches and the importance of inclusivity, diversity, and informed decision-making.

She also highlighted the fact that investigational treatments were not yet approved for human use so, in effect, could actually be harmful until proven otherwise which reinforced the idea that her role was to protect patients as much as possible when they were, after all, putting their health, and possibly lives, at risk by participating in a clinical trial.

Another element Dr. Mitchell was keen to emphasize was the level of expertise among the members of the Ethics Committee. She pointed out that many of them had 'seen and heard it all' and that one of their primary concerns was to ensure that a trial was fit for purpose.

Josh, eager to gain further clarity, posed a series of pertinent questions to Dr. Mitchell, seeking to understand the intricacies of the EC's role in patient recruitment.

"Dr. Mitchell, could you provide us with insights into the specific materials or documents that an EC reviews in the context of patient recruitment? Are there any particular aspects or criteria that you consider when evaluating these?" Josh asked.

"Certainly, Josh. As I've already said, when it comes to patient recruitment, the EC or IRB typically reviews and assesses all the various documentation involved and any other materials that may be used to engage potential participants – sometimes with 'everything but the kitchen sink' being thrown at us for review, which does place something of a burden on us to do our jobs thoroughly" Dr. Mitchell explained.

Max couldn't help but add a sardonic comment. "Well, in my experience it often seems like the IRB's main job is to make sure no patients are recruited rather than merely protecting them from being coerced."

"I can appreciate your perspective, Max. However, it's important to understand that the EC's or IRB's primary goal is to ensure the protection and well-being of trial participants," Dr. Mitchell replied. "While it may sometimes feel like there are stringent requirements and meticulous scrutiny, it's essential to remember that the EC's role is to balance scientific progress with ethical considerations and the potential implications of what is being said. Our aim is to safeguard participants from undue harm and ensure that they make informed decisions about their involvement in clinical trials. For example, direct advertising can be viewed from a regulatory perspective as the start of the informed consent process – so we have to be strict with what can and can't be said in order to ensure patients are given the right information to make the choice that's right for them."

Josh wanted to share the thought that had been brewing in his mind. "Dr. Mitchell, it seems to me that closer collaboration among the various stakeholders, particularly bringing patients into the fold, could be a valuable approach," he said. "And by involving patients in trial design, recruitment strategies, and even marketing efforts, we have an opportunity to create a more patient-centric approach that addresses their needs and concerns."

Dr. Mitchell responded warmly. "I appreciate your perspective, Josh. Patient involvement at every stage of the process can indeed lead to more meaningful and patient-centered trials," she affirmed. "By fostering collaboration, listening to patients' voices, and valuing their experiences, we can help to collectively shape the clinical trials landscape to better serve the needs of those who participate. Not to mention the fact that involving members of the public and trial participants is set to become mandatory – something that I for one hope will help us in our goal of increased diversity.

And, of course, there's the issue of expanded access for people who sometimes literally have nowhere else to go. Allowing these people to have an investigational treatment prior to it being approved is another complex issue that requires careful handling to ensure patients understand the risks involved."

Josh and Max exchanged glances. Josh was starting to believe that the path to improving patient recruitment and retention lay in collaborative efforts, breaking down silos, and placing patients alongside the other stakeholders at the heart of the decision-making process.

As the meeting drew to a close, the thorny issues of payments for trial participants and data privacy also having reared their head, Josh thanked Dr. Mitchell for her time and the valuable input she had given.

"Any closer to solving the puzzle, do you think?" Max asked Josh, teeing-up their next meeting.

Josh nodded, and replied "Indeed I think we're getting closer, Max. Now let's see what we can learn from someone who thinks they might already have the solution to the problem.

Chapter Seventeen – The Patient Recruitment Vendor

Max clicked through to the next meeting and joined the video call. As he did so, a face familiar to him appeared on the screen – Hank Davidson, the brash and assertive representative of the patient recruitment vendor.

Hank, a middle-aged American with a charismatic presence, oozed confidence and spoke with an air of self-assuredness. His boisterous demeanor was matched by his quick wit and an unmistakable twinkle in the eye. Hank had carved a reputation in the industry for his no-nonsense approach and a track record of delivering results – including having worked on several trials for Awex when Max was involved there.

Josh was prepared for Hank's spirited personality having heard of his reputation from Max. With the introductory pleasantries out of the way, Josh started the conversational ball rolling.

"Hank," he said, "could you give us with some details about how your firm goes about recruiting patients? Specifically, I'm interested in understanding how you utilize digital outreach, and the results you typically see from these campaigns."

Hank leaned back in his chair, a confident smile gracing his face. He was more than happy to share his expertise. "Well, guys, let me tell you, digital outreach has been a game-changer when it comes to patient recruitment. We primarily leverage platforms like Facebook Ads to reach a wide audience and engage potential participants.

Through targeted campaigns and personalized messaging, we can capture the attention of individuals who may be eligible for clinical trials. We utilize sophisticated algorithms and data analytics to optimize our ads to ensure they're reaching the right people at the right time."

Max nodded in agreement, as Hank leaned forward, his eyes gleaming with excitement. "You might not believe it Josh but, as I'm sure Max can testify, digital outreach campaigns, particularly through platforms like Facebook, often account for 60% or more of the patients recruited into trials. The power of digital advertising when wielded effectively is truly remarkable," he emphasized.

Max nodded again. However, ever keen to inject some irony into proceedings, he responded. "So, Hank, you're telling us that Facebook Ads are the secret weapon for patient recruitment? Who would've thought?" he quipped.

Hank chuckled. "Well, Max, it may sound simple but, when it comes to reaching potential participants efficiently and effectively, digital outreach is truly a powerful tool. Of course, it requires expertise, data-driven strategies, and continuous optimization but the results – as you well know from your previous dealings with us – speak for themselves," he replied.

Hank went on to outline the process in detail, talking Josh and Max through the various stages of developing and executing a successful digital outreach campaign for patient recruitment.

He began by explaining the initial steps involved in creating a compelling digital ad and an engaging landing page. Hank stressed the importance of crafting targeted messaging that would resonate with the intended audience and designing a user-friendly landing page that would encourage potential patients to take action – incorporating elements of pre-screening to ensure the applicants were likely to fit the eligibility criteria for the trial.

Continuing, Hank delved into the regulatory aspects of the process. He described the meticulous review and approval process that digital ads and landing pages underwent by IRBs/ECs – as Josh and Max had recently been hearing from Dr. Mitchell. He highlighted the need to adhere to these ethical guidelines, ensuring that the materials provided accurate and transparent information about the clinical trial, as well as pointing out that the various digital platforms had guidelines of their own that need to be considered.

Hank then explained how the campaign unfolded from the moment a potential patient clicked on the ad and arrived at the landing page. He discussed the significance of capturing their interest and encouraging them to provide their contact details. This, he explained, allowed for a follow-up call to confirm the applicant's eligibility and to arrange a visit with the research site.

He outlined some of the common payment models for patient recruitment vendors – ranging from the agency-style model of a fixed fee for hourly input into the campaigns, through a pay per lead model and to the model that Hank's firm primarily used – pay per patient. Hank was scathing of the pay per lead model as operated by some firms in the industry, suggesting it was one of the main reasons the research sites did not like central ad campaigns, as an unscrupulous vendor would be paid even for low quality leads.

Josh, always seeking deeper understanding, posed pertinent questions, exploring the nuances of the process. He asked about the effectiveness of sites following up with patients to arrange their own initial screening visits, and whether this posed challenges.

Hank did not hold back, sharing his candid perspective.

"You know, Josh, it's one of the big drawbacks we often face. While the digital outreach campaigns are effective in attracting potential patients, the responsibility of arranging the visits usually falls on the research sites which almost always leads to delays and inefficiencies as sites may have limited resources or face difficulties in scheduling appointments," Hank responded.

Max, in agreement with Hank's observation, chimed in. "Ah, the classic bottleneck of site-level coordination. Seems like it's a hurdle that many face," he remarked.

Hank nodded in agreement. "You've hit the nail on the head, Max. It's an ongoing challenge, but one that we're constantly working to address. Collaboration and streamlining processes between patient recruitment vendors, sites, and trial sponsors are something that I for one consider to be the key to overcoming these obstacles," he added.

Josh, intrigued by Hank's insights, posed a question that delved into exploring potential support methods for the digital outreach approach taken by Hank's firm.

"Hank, based on your experience, what do you think would be a beneficial support method for the digital outreach approach your firm employs?" Josh asked.

"A good start would be the sites using some of the solutions that already exist to help to improve the conversion rate from application to screening visit," Hank replied. "It would certainly make for a more effective process if we could allow patients to book their own visits. Or even have the people who make any follow-up calls able to schedule the appointments at the site."

"And any other factors you think would help improve results?" Josh asked.

"Well," Hank replied, "I'm sure you've already been made aware that some of the inclusion/exclusion criteria for modern clinical trials are somewhat restrictive."

Josh and Max both smiled and nodded.

"And the choice of sites made in the feasibility and selection process can also be a bit limiting," Hank went on, "with our targeting being forced to aim for very small areas that might not have especially large populations.

But one of the other things I think the industry could do to improve things from our perspective is to enhance its reputation. Anyone who promotes a clinical trial using a social media advert will have seen people commenting with phrases such as 'guinea pig' which I assume is likely to put some people off who might otherwise have considered applying. Maybe having more of an understanding within society as a whole of the benefits of clinical trials could help to encourage more acceptance of it being vital for advancing medicine."

Josh could see the logic in this and as the meeting with Hank drew to a close, Josh and Max expressed their gratitude, thanking him for his valuable insights and the engaging discussion. They concluded the video call on a positive note, appreciative of the knowledge gained from their conversation.

Josh and Max took a moment to reflect on their learnings then Josh said "Max, given we've spoken to various different stakeholders in the process, I think we should also have a conversation with a primary care provider. I think we need to gain insights into their perspectives and understand any barriers they may encounter in recommending trials to their patients," he suggested.

Max nodded in agreement. "Absolutely, Black. Gaining first-hand insights from doctors will help us to uncover the underlying reasons behind why they don't traditionally refer all that many patients into trials. It's essential to understand their perspective to create meaningful solutions," he replied.

They decided to take a break and satiate their hunger with a visit to the hotel restaurant for lunch, and made their way to the inviting eatery, a relaxed ambiance providing the ideal backdrop for their post-meeting review discussion during which Max announced that their next activity had already been arranged. Apparently, this could incorporate meeting a primary care practitioner and should certainly yield some additional insights for Josh in his puzzle-solving quest.

"Great," Josh said, "where is it we're going?"

"Vegas, baby!" Max responded, somewhat surprising Josh mid-mouthful such that he nearly dropped his fork.

Max continued. "We'll be leaving this evening on an overnight flight then a couple of days from now we're attending a conference for people who work in clinical operations – one that attracts many of the relevant stakeholders when it comes to patient recruitment. In fact, I should think Hank's firm will be represented – maybe by the man himself."

Josh smiled. He had been to Las Vegas a few times and always enjoyed it so immediately started to look forward to the next stage of the journey.

Chapter Eighteen – The Only Way to Travel

Josh was not surprised that Max – through Alexander Wexford's office – had booked them in first class. He wondered if it was the norm for the industry to experience the best that travel had to offer. Or if it was just something that happened after selling your company for hundreds of millions of dollars. Whichever it was, he wasn't about to start complaining!

They had enjoyed the hospitality in the exclusive lounge and because it was an evening flight, they were served an evening meal that was apparently based on suggestions from one of the world's leading chefs.

It was certainly a far cry from the experience Josh had first had flying to Las Vegas for a friend's bachelor party (known as a 'stag do' in the UK) back when he was in his early twenties.

After finishing their meals, Josh and Max met up in the socializing bar area of the first class cabin.

"Enjoy your meal, Black?" Max asked, already a step ahead of Josh with two glasses of champagne on the table in front of him.

"Indeed I did, Max," Josh replied, "indeed I did."

He sat down and joined in the champagne toast.

"To Alexander Wexford," Max said.

"And solving puzzles," Josh replied.

They both smiled and settled into a conversation about where they had been, and what they had to look forward to through the rest of their quest – Max updating Josh with details of what he might expect at the conference they would be attending in a day or so.

Once they had got through their discussion on the matter at hand, Josh asked Max about the 'Rock the Blues' musical he had seen in London.

"Ah, the show was an absolute blast," Max exclaimed. "I've always been a huge blues rock fan – especially from the classic era of the sixties and seventies – so it was right up my alley."

He went on to describe some of the standout performances and memorable moments from the show. Max's expressive gestures and vivid descriptions brought the energy and excitement of the musical to life, transporting Josh into the world of dazzling lights and toe-tapping rhythms.

As Josh sipped his champagne and got caught up in the enthusiasm of his companion, the melody he had heard Max whistling yesterday came back to him so he asked if it was in the show.

"Oh yes," Max replied. "That was the big finale. There's a few versions of that song but my favorite's the one by Canned Heat. And actually it seems rather appropriate for what we're trying to achieve."

Josh was intrigued but also tired by now so they bid each other good night and retreated to the individual flatbed seating pods – shutting out the cabin around them as they hurtled across the Atlantic at 600 miles per hour.

Chapter Nineteen – Vegas Villa

Josh had anticipated staying at the conference hotel but Max disabused him of this idea once they landed at Harry Reid International, Vegas's main airport.

"Well, Black," Max informed him, "Alexander Wexford owns a villa near The Strip so whenever anyone from Awex came to Vegas, they stayed there. As we are going to do."

The pre-booked limousine whisked them away from the airport, taking in the sights on The Strip, then turning off to the east along Sands Avenue. Max explained the location of the villa was ideal, being approximately a ten minute walk from The Strip and the hotel where the conference was being held.

Once again, Josh found himself comparing this experience with his previous visits – some of which had certainly been more extravagant than others but none of which were likely to match up to the kind of thing that Alexander Wexford might be able to lay on.

Once inside the villa – a uniformed butler having opened the door for them – Josh marveled at the size of the place, and the seemingly authentic original artworks on the walls.

"The Bellagio and Wynn hotels have quite a few original pieces," Max said, inspecting one of the paintings more closely, "so I should think this place is only third on the list of LV vacation residences that host fine artworks."

Josh was further impressed as the butler – an Englishman in his mid-thirties who introduced himself only as 'Evans' – showed him to his room. Having thought the hotel suite in London was quite luxurious, Josh was pleased to see the Sin City version of his accommodation was no less well-appointed.

Evans indicated he would unpack Josh's suitcase then led him out to the backyard pool – a large complex of inter-connected pools, fountains, and hot tub areas where Josh and Max were presented with more champagne and a selection of canapes.

"I tell you what, Max," Josh said, relaxing into a sun lounger. "For an industry that gets something so fundamentally wrong about one of its core activities, there certainly seems to be a lot of upside still available in terms of the money to be made."

Max chuckled in agreement, clinked his glass on Josh's, and turned his eyes to the setting sun.

Chapter Twenty – The Clinical Trials Conference

The rest of the day went by very pleasantly, the only work-related talk being of when they would be leaving the next day for the conference.

Next morning, at the appointed hour, the same black limousine that had brought them from the airport turned up at the villa to transport them to their destination.

"I thought it was only a ten minute walk," Josh said, causing Max to laugh.

"It is," he replied, "but in 95-degree heat – something like 35 in European money, I believe – you'll be glad of the air conditioning."

He was right. The blast of warm air that greeted them as they stepped outside was sufficient to make Josh realise a ten minute walk in that kind of weather would certainly have left him feeling uncomfortable, especially in the suit he was wearing.

On arrival at the conference venue – one of the mega hotels that Las Vegas specializes in – Max registered them both and picked up their lanyards. Josh could not help but notice they both said 'Gold VIP Access all Areas' – another testament to Alexander Wexford's retained status within the industry.

Max was greeted warmly by the conference organizer – a veteran of these events, with many successful conferences under his belt, and a man known as a super connector who knew just about everyone in the industry.

"No agenda?" Josh asked, looking for details on what was coming up – once again causing Max to chuckle.

"Not a printed one, grandad," he replied, using his phone to scan a QR code on the registration desk which downloaded the conference's digital agenda.

Josh did the same then looked through the sessions that were coming up over the next few days. The conference started with a keynote from a world-renowned author of multiple best-selling books in the popular science genre then had different tracks that could be followed depending on one's interests.

Max pointed out a few sessions he suggested they attend then highlighted some of the names of the people they should speak to.

"At the same time, Black," he elaborated, "there'll be lots to glean from the vendors in the exhibition hall. Looks like that opens after lunch today so will be well worth a visit. And don't go imagining you'll be able to get round it all today. There are so many firms here it'll be worth our while doing the rounds every day to get as much as we can from them."

Josh was a little surprised by this but on looking at the list of exhibitors, he realized there were over 200 of them so indeed it would be impossible to get round them all in an afternoon.

"Of course, some of them aren't worth bothering with," Max went on. "But we won't really know that until we take a closer look."

As they fueled-up on coffee and biscuits, ready for the morning's sessions, Max pointed out some familiar faces in the milling throng –

some of whom waved and smiled at him while others ignored him, already deep in conversation with colleagues and acquaintances.

"Now, Black," Max said, "one thing you need to know about these conferences – you could easily come away thinking the industry is doing fine as it is, with everybody working towards the same common goals. But the big problems are, either everyone here is already so in tune with doing things the right way that they may as well be preaching to the converted, or everyone goes away wanting to implement everything they've learned, then promptly gets caught up in day-to-day stuff and forgets about it within a week."

Josh took this in and continued reading the agenda. There was one particular track he was drawn to – Decentralized Trials (DCTs). He had read and heard quite a lot about these but only really in passing with no proper understanding of what they were or how they were supposed to work.

"Well if it's DCTs you're interested in, Black," Max informed him, "as indeed you very well should be, there's no need to get the lowdown from me that I promised you – you should speak to Bob Simons. He's one of the founding fathers of the whole movement. And you can be sure he's here – he'd go to the opening of an envelope if he thought there were photographers around."

Max searched through the agenda on his phone and pointed out the multiple sessions that featured Bob Simons – either in conversation with a questioner or as a discussion panelist. He highlighted a particular session that was due that morning just before the mid-morning break.

"That's our chance," he said. "If we hang around long enough after that session, we'll be able to collar him for a private chat."

Josh looked quizzical about the possibility of that happening with so many other attendees being around but Max simply put his index finger to the side of his nose, saying "Don't you worry about that, Black. Even if my name doesn't carry all that much weight anymore, you can be sure that Alexander's does."

Chapter Twenty-one – The Decentralized Trials Evangelist

The first three sessions of the morning had come to a close – Josh having learned more than he ever expected about how big pharma companies were supposedly embracing the patient engagement movement and how the whole industry now had diversity, equity, and inclusion running through its core.

Max hurried him from where they were sitting to a huddle of people gathered around the most recent session's main guest, Bob Simons. Max and Bob did a 'bro nod' as they caught sight of each other while Bob continued talking.

After a minute or two, Bob thanked the others for their interest, telling them he had a prior meeting booked that he now had to get off to. At this, Josh was a little crestfallen at first until he realized the meeting Bob was talking about was with him and Max.

"Donovan, how nice to see you," Bob said, extending his hand in greeting. "And who's your unusual friend?"

It took Josh a second to realize Bob Simons was talking about him. 'Unusual?'

Max laughed and grasped Bob's hand warmly. "Marvelous to see you, too, Simons. This is Josh Black – the famous puzzle-solving podcaster."

Bob eyed him with a respectful expression on his face.

"And what he means by unusual, Black," Max said, "is that he hasn't met you before. Those of us who have, know how unusual you really are but don't worry – it doesn't show to those who haven't."

Max and Bob both laughed at Max's joke – perhaps a bit too much for Josh's taste, but he smiled along with them and also shook Bob's hand.

"A pleasure to meet you, Mr. Simons," Josh said, causing both Max and Bob to burst out laughing again.

"It's either Simons or Bob," Bob replied, shaking Josh's hand. "Mr. Simons is my father. God rest his soul. Now then, Donovan," he continued, turning to face Max, "what brings a millionaire ex-employee of Alexander Wexford to this kind of jamboree? Trying to stir up trouble, as usual?"

Max smiled and explained what they were doing, and how they were interested in hearing more about DCTs 'from the horse's mouth'. Bob Simons said he would be speaking at the next session but for the next fifteen minutes he could chat with them in one of the breakout rooms so he could tell them all about it.

"So," he began, once the three of them were sitting around the room's small desk, "what have you heard about decentralized trials and their relationship to patient recruitment?"

Max allowed Josh to answer. "As far as I know, it's a concept that brings the clinical trial experience directly to the patients, often leveraging technology to facilitate remote participation away from the confines of the traditional research site" he replied.

Bob nodded. "Absolutely, Black. Decentralized trials have the potential to address many of the challenges the industry has encountered in recruiting patients. By incorporating digital platforms, wearable tech, and telemedicine, patients can participate in trials from the comfort of their own homes, eliminating the need for frequent site visits," he said. "But it's about more than just technology, it's about using new and innovative methods to enable patients to take part in trials without having to attend a site to do so – essentially being more about process than about technology."

"Fair enough, "Josh replied. But there are some specific tech solutions I keep hearing about – such as electronic consent. Is this the kind of thing that would be included as DCT?"

"Yes," Bob replied, "and yet so much more. Econsent and ePRO – that's Patient Reported Outcomes – would certainly fall within the parameters of DCT. As would such things as home visits by people working on the study, virtual visits which can be done online, visits that the patient can make to non-site venues, and possibly even having the investigational treatment delivered directly to a patient's home, if desired.

Everything is designed to make the process as easy as possible for someone to participate in a trial, as well as making life easier for those people operating the trial. Though you might not think so from some of the reactions we get from people at the traditional research sites. I think they fear they'll be burdened with yet more tech to learn – when actually if done properly, with proper training, resources, and compensation provided, DCT solutions can be a benefit to any site."

Max added, "And let's not forget about mobile research sites. These mobile units can travel to communities and reach underserved populations, making it more convenient for patients to participate in trials which can be a great way to bring trials closer to the patients, breaking down geographical barriers."

Bob chimed in. "Absolutely, Donovan. Mobile research sites not only increase access to trials but also provide a familiar and comfortable environment for patients, fostering trust and participation. It's an interesting solution that addresses the challenge of reaching diverse patient populations which, as we all know, is a major thing for the industry at the moment," he said. "And on the same theme, if only we could get them more interested, it could well be that we can get local primary care providers to help out. The technology already exists for them to simply provide the space and a nurse with remote and virtual monitoring for ongoing visits by someone off-site."

Josh picked up the idea. "I've heard of some trials that have leveraged retail pharmacies for clinical trial solutions," he said. "I believe the idea is that, as with doctors, many pharmacies already have established relationships with patients and by offering trials within their premises, they can expand patient recruitment efforts and create a more accessible pathway for participation."

Bob did not seem too enthusiastic about this, but grudgingly appeared to agree. "You're maybe onto something, Black. Pharmacies have a wide network and frequent foot traffic which obviously would provide an opportunity to engage with potential trial participants and raise awareness about the benefits of clinical trials," he acknowledged. "But it appears that, post-Covid, some of the major pharmacies may be getting cold feet about the idea though there are still some who remain committed to their various projects, which again helps with the underlying goal of providing choice for patients.

Fundamentally, the whole raison d'etre of DCTs is about focusing on flexibility, choice, and providing options for trial participants.

We're certainly not there yet, but I'm determined to help get us there in the end."

As they continued their discussion, exploring the possibilities of decentralized trials, Josh could understand the enthusiasm that Bob had for DCTs but wondered if there was something missing in the approach that many solutions providers were taking.

"So, it appears to me," he said, not wishing to sound confrontational, "that the majority of DCT solutions – at least the ones I've seen so far – are purely tech-based. But doesn't that somehow miss out on the essential human element required to reassure patients their needs are being looked after?"

Bob leant forward, folding his arms on the desk. "Don't imagine, Josh," he said, for once using Josh's first name, "that just because I'm a DCT evangelist, I agree with everything that might be put forward in its name."

He checked his watch before continuing solemnly. "It may certainly appear as if DCT solutions are all about the tech but myself, and many others, are working towards a future where the tech is used for what it is – a shining beacon of hope amongst the myriad lesser options. A towering testament to the power of human thought and the genius of those involved in its development. A solution like no other to the problems facing humanity."

Josh was a little taken aback by how portentous Bob had sounded then noticed the smile appearing at the corners of his mouth before both Bob and Max burst out laughing.

"Anyway," Bob went on, "while I may be exaggerating for comedic effect, the basic idea remains the same. Tech plus human input is the way forward for DCTs, rather than it being an end in its own right. And with that, gentleman – and Donovan – I have to be getting to my next session."

Chapter Twenty-two – The Patient Recruitment Consultant

In between the sessions Max had highlighted as being worth attending, he and Josh spent a lot of time reviewing the vendor booths in the exhibition hall. There they found all manner of solutions providers offering an extraordinary range of different products and services to help with the clinical trials process.

They tried to focus primarily on the booths related to patient recruitment with many specialist vendors having their own approach to the problem, one of which was Hank Davidson's firm, who had taken out a spectacular booth that was attracting a lot of attention. Hank waved at them, gesturing to all the people around him as if to say he would love to chat but was too busy. Josh and Max smiled, waved back, and continued their tour of the hall.

"Max Donovan!" came a cultured-sounding English voice. Josh turned to see an extremely good-looking blond-haired man of indeterminate age – one of the only people in the conference venue to be wearing a tie.

"Russ Johnson!" Max replied, hugging the man warmly. Josh could not help but notice that lots of other people were also greeting this man with affection as they stopped to say hello.

"Black, meet Russ Johnson, a fellow Englishman if you hadn't guessed," Max said by way of introduction. "Probably the most charming, witty, and charismatic fellow you could hope to meet. And something of a legend when it comes to patient recruitment."

"Well, I try my best," Russ replied. "Nice to meet you Mr. Black," he continued, extending his hand.

Josh took the handshake, replying, "Josh, please."

They spent a minute or two with Max and Russ catching up on a few things then arranged to meet up later for a proper chat over a few drinks.

Josh was intrigued by Russ Johnson. If he was a patient recruitment expert, why hadn't Alexander Wexford and Max Donovan invited him to participate in the project?

During a coffee break later that day, Josh checked out Russ's LinkedIn profile and found a wealth of short videos and articles relating to patient recruitment and retention as well as links to a couple of books he had written on the subject. In these, Russ often put forward the idea that there were two primary issues in patient recruitment – lack of awareness that trials exist, plus lack of access for patients who may wish to take part, and five key elements to any patient recruitment strategy – finding, engaging, qualifying, consenting, and retaining.

It seemed like he would be the ideal candidate to pursue the project he and Max were working on so Josh asked Max about it once he had picked up his own coffee.

"Ah, that's a good question," Max replied. "And actually, the answer is that we did approach him some time ago to help us with our own issues. Back when we were still with Awex. And he did help us out a lot with many of our active projects but, when it came to this idea, he told us he'd have to think about it then eventually recommended we approach you instead."

Josh was shocked. "Really?" he spluttered, almost spitting out a mouthful of coffee. "Why would he do that?"

"Why don't you ask him yourself? We're meeting with him in an hour or so," Max replied.

The rest of the afternoon was filled with sessions and quick conversations with vendors and people who Max knew from his previous role. All the while Josh was wondering if there was something he was missing about the project he was working on that had caused one of the world's leading consultants in the field to request his involvement.

As their get-together drew near, Josh could not help but feel both pride in the fact that his own efforts had been recognized as potentially being useful, and apprehension as to what Russ Johnson might say.

"Max, my man," Josh heard Russ say as they approached him at a bar room table, "I've already got the first round in. Thought we'd start with a nice Chablis then move on from there. What do you think, Josh?"

"Sounds good to me," Josh replied, settling into a comfortable seat at the table and accepting the proffered glass.

"Now then, Russ," Max said – Josh noticing he was not using the consultant's surname, "Josh here has a question for you."

Josh gulped his first mouthful of wine and asked why he had been brought into the project.

"Quite simple, really," Russ replied. "I thought you could help."

Russ drained his glass, topped it up and continued. "It's often the case that people from other disciplines can spot things that people who are already immersed in what they're doing maybe can't. Happens quite frequently in art – for example Picasso with his experimental ceramics. And it occurred to me that someone who's adept at solving puzzles, but not necessarily familiar with the world of clinical trials, would be perfect to take on the challenge suggested by Alexander Wexford."

Russ took a further sip and went on. "I've listened to all of your podcasts, Josh, and think you're something of a genius when it comes to putting the pieces of a puzzle together in innovative ways."

Josh could not help but smile at that, holding his own glass to his lips slightly longer than usual to try to curb any outward signs of his growing embarrassment.

"And I've tried to emulate your techniques myself when looking at the problems of patient recruitment," Russ went on, "but with only limited success which is why I thought there's no point me trying to do the work of the master when the master might be available to do it himself."

Josh could understand why Max had described this guy as being charming and charismatic, and found himself listening intently as Russ carried on.

"I particularly liked your explanation of how to use inversion when studying a problem," Russ said. "And applied it myself to the area of patient recruitment. Now, I'm sure you've probably already done this, but if you'll allow me to give you a quick outline of what I believe a patient recruitment and retention project would look like if it was set up to fail?"

Josh smiled and nodded for Russ to carry on.

"Thanks. Well, let's see, first of all, you'd make sure nobody could find out about the project. There are obviously ethics regulations to be followed, so you'd upload it to the relevant place but outside of that you'd have no online presence for the trial, and no other promotional material.

But even before that, of course, at the stage where you're designing the trial, you'd make the qualification procedure so strict that almost nobody would qualify in the first place. And even if someone does, in order to make sure they wouldn't be interested in taking part, you'd design the protocol without asking for any input from patients or the research sites who are likely to be operating the trial."

Josh continued smiling along. He could tell Russ was getting more animated and venting his frustrations on all that was wrong with patient recruitment.

"Next," he continued, "you'd choose only research sites that had no existing patients with the condition you were testing a potential treatment for. And, for good measure, you'd make them very inaccessible even to those people who might qualify and wish to take part.

Talking of which, you'd offer no incentive of any kind to the trial participants, and precious little to anyone else who might want to attract patients to take part such as the research sites. And, obviously, you'd choose a huge global CRO to set everything up and manage it on your behalf, but only so long as they would refuse to enlist the help of any patient recruitment solutions providers.

And if, by some miracle, you did manage to recruit enough patients in the first place, you'd ensure that not enough of them remained on the trial to completion by making the burden of participation extremely onerous, treating them very badly, keeping them in the dark about progress, and essentially making it clear that they were just a very small cog in the overall machine and it didn't really matter whether they were involved or not."

Max started laughing and interjected, "yes indeed. No point giving the patients any ideas that they might actually be the most important element in the whole process."

Russ and Josh both smiled, each taking a sip of their newly replenished glasses.

"I don't think I need go on any further," Russ said, "but I'd also ensure no doctors were encouraged to discuss the trial, no community organizations were approached to promote it. And, as an additional failsafe, that there was no thought for any long-term relationship building that might help with future trial recruitment."

Josh clapped his hands together, saying "well that certainly sums up how I was thinking about the inversion process, thank you."

"No, thank you," Russ responded. "If you can genuinely come up with a possible solution – or range of solutions, I guess – to improve the situation, the world will certainly be a better place. Well, at least the world of clinical trials, at least."

They all laughed and clinked glasses together, Max gesturing to a nearby waiter that they would like another bottle.

"Of course," Russ went on, "if you actually wanted to do a good job, you might consider utilizing a network of sites that can take advantage of each other's databases. And if you can arrange it so any follow-up call that's necessary in the application process happens quickly, and is handled by people with medical training, that will also help with having everything run smoothly.

And just to emphasize again the importance of the burden of taking part in a trial. I've always considered that, on a hot day, no amount of marketing fluff will work better for a café than to simply put up a sign saying 'free ice cream'. Making the product – the trial itself – more attractive could help win half the battle when it comes to attracting participants."

Josh nodded and asked Russ directly "I think it's interesting you mentioned doctors earlier, Russ – we've been thinking of talking with some, so do you think primary care physicians should be a valuable source of patients for trials?"

"Should be," Russ responded, "but sadly rarely are. There's a whole delegation of them here if you want to get their thoughts on the matter."

Josh agreed this would be a good idea and Max set himself the task of arranging a meet with some primary care doctors during the conference.

The conversation continued, covering recruiting patients for different types of trial – including observational trials that may be based on analyzing data from the past, or from following a group of participants over time, plus ongoing trials of such things as wellness apps, or looking at the effect of non-clinical activities like eating five pieces of fruit a day.

Russ also touched on the fact that, while translating patient recruitment materials to target non-English speakers is fairly routine for campaigns in primarily non-English speaking countries, it could also make sense in places like the UK and USA where a significant number of people have English as their second language. He also mentioned the potential success to be had from utilizing influencers, or Key Opinion Leaders, for promoting trials. And how combining these two elements – translation plus influence – can be especially beneficial.

"And now, gentlemen," Russ said during a suitable pause in their discussion, "while this sort of thing is effectively what we're here for, it might be time to forget our day jobs for a while and have a more convivial conversation. What do you say?"

Josh and Max agreed, and the three of them spent the next few hours enjoying each other's company being joined at regular intervals by people in the bar who recognized Russ, Max, or both, and wanted to make sure they came to say hello.

Chapter Twenty-three – The Primary Care Physicians

Next morning – well, it was still just about morning when Josh was able to make it down from his room – Max had arranged a meeting with two doctors, one from the UK and one from the US.

Josh had assumed their experiences would be quite dissimilar with the two healthcare systems being based on very different payment models but actually it appeared there were more similarities than he would have thought.

Dr. Emma Fitzgerald was the UK doctor, Dr. Ben Cohn from the US.

Dr. Fitzgerald outlined some of the issues they faced. "The demands of providing comprehensive care within limited appointment slots can be overwhelming. It's a constant juggling act to address patients' immediate concerns, diagnose ailments, and discuss suitable treatments, all while ensuring their well-being."

Dr. Cohn nodded in empathy.

She continued, her frustration apparent. "Remembering to consider clinical trial opportunities for each patient within such brief consultations becomes increasingly challenging. It's not just a matter of time, but also the mental workload of keeping up with current trials, eligibility criteria, and research protocols."

Dr. Cohn added "I want what's best for my patients, and clinical trials can hold promise for innovative treatments and advancements. However, the sheer volume of information we need to process in a limited timeframe often leaves little room to explore potential trial opportunities so I'm mostly unaware that relevant trials might exist."

Dr. Fitzgerald chimed in again. "I also want to emphasize that not all patients are suitable candidates for clinical trials, and not all clinical trials are suitable to test on all patients," she stated firmly. "Clinical trials are a critical part of advancing medical knowledge and developing new treatments, but we must remember that treatments undergoing trial are essentially unproven substances. They may hold promise but until they have been rigorously tested for safety and efficacy, they carry inherent risks."

Dr. Cohn took up the theme. "As healthcare providers, our utmost priority is the well-being and safety of our patients. While clinical trials offer potential benefits, they also involve uncertainties and potential side effects. It's our responsibility to carefully evaluate each patient's specific circumstances, taking into account their medical history, current condition, and the risks and benefits associated with participation in a particular trial."

Josh understood this perspective, and wanted to learn more about an issue they had heard about affecting US doctors.

"So, Dr. Cohn," he asked, "is it true that doctors in the US are afraid they might lose their patient to a rival doctor if they put them forward for a clinical trial?"

"It may be the case for some, yes," Dr. Cohn replied, "but it's not something I'd be especially concerned about myself. And I know it's not going to be an issue for Emma, as obviously the NHS works quite differently. But for me, the main issue isn't losing the patient who, after all, can be replaced anyway."

Max interjected "and I believe there are multiple solutions nowadays that we might label DCT that would enable a doctor to keep their patient while still having them participate in a different doctor's trial."

"Indeed that's true, Max," Dr. Cohn responded, "though we're something of a slow-moving industry, you might have noticed, so not everyone will be as forward-looking as to consider that option. But the main issue for me – even if I do want to inform patients about a trial – is the timing of when I do so. It's a common occurrence for me to mention a particular disease or ailment, and notice the patient's brain is then completely absorbed with the implications of that so they're unable to take in anything else."

Dr. Fitzgerald agreed "that's definitely my experience too," she said. "And in all the years I've been practising medicine, I've never come across a better way to inform a patient than to come straight out with it."

Josh thought for a moment, then said "so ideally the time to mention a clinical trial isn't necessarily at the point of telling the person their diagnosis, but at some future stage?"

"Or tell them at the point of diagnosis," Dr. Cohn said, "and then remind them at a future stage."

They continued for another few minutes, touching on the small but significant level of success each had seen through having clinical trials promoted in their waiting rooms on TV sets or through having leaflets readily available. Both also agreeing that the idea of having primary care physicians refer patients for clinical trials was a good one but that it was unlikely to work all that well in the current way of doing things.

Josh and Max thanked the two doctors for their input, and made their way back to the conference exhibit hall to explore more of the solutions on offer.

Chapter Twenty-four – The Elevator Pitch Solution

While walking around the booths and exhibits, Josh got the feeling that the majority of solutions providers were looking at things from a technical perspective. Seemingly every other vendor had incorporated an AI element into their solution – some of which appeared to make sense, others of which appeared to be a solution in search of a problem.

One area that did look promising was the speeding up of the chart review process to identify patients who might be suitable for specific trials. Josh found out from several vendor representatives that done manually, the process could take several hours, and even days, before a suitable number of potential candidates was found by sifting through their records.

Josh had spoken with representatives of patient databases – from labs and other organizations – who could provide direct access to healthcare professionals and sometimes patients themselves who had perhaps had a recent diagnosis of a relevant condition.

Methods had been demonstrated for giving patients better access to information about trials. Max explained to Josh that very few people were actively seeking a trial to take part in but, for those who were, the main government-agency databases were unwieldy and difficult to navigate. Bringing a better user experience to this process – also with medical speak translated into a layperson's language – was one of the core benefits of these new approaches.

Josh had also seen firms offering solutions such as providing gifts to patients at various stages – backpacks, mouse mats etc. – as a means of retaining them on a trial, plus some solutions that incorporated elements of 'gamification' into taking part – for example achieving different levels of the 'game' for each time some Patient Reported Outcomes were uploaded into the system.

Methods of easing the patient burden were on display – including such things as concierge-style services that dealt with transport and accommodation for trial participants who lived away from the research site they were attending.

Various other solutions were on offer for having duplicate patients – in a virtual sense – and constructing a trial based purely on computer modeling. Meanwhile, others were based on trying to link up the whole health care ecosystem such that every visit to a doctor, every visit to a research site, every visit to a hospital etc., was recorded and the data centralized in such a way that it could be utilized for the benefit of both society as a whole, and each person whose data was being recorded.

This was an idea that fascinated Josh. Having been born in the UK, he had assumed there was a central database that held all his NHS records from birth that could be accessed by other health care professionals within the same system. However, that was far from being the case – even in this digital age.

From a purely patient recruitment perspective, this kind of centralized big data should allow for a much quicker method of identifying and communicating with potential trial participants. 'Maybe someday,' Josh thought, deciding he wanted to go to the business lounge in the hotel for a short time to gather his thoughts.

Max was on his way to an upstairs meeting room when Josh got to the elevator. On stepping into the not quite crowded space, Max started with his trademark humor.

"They say elevators are the perfect place for networking," he said. "So, what's your pitch? Mine's 'I'm Max, and I can make any awkward elevator ride hilarious.'"

There were a few nervous giggles before Max spoke again.

"Well, I guess that kind of reaction is just part of the ups and downs of elevator life," he said, generating a few more giggles from the other occupants.

"And with all these 'e's being prefixed to so many of the solutions on offer, I started to think I was back in the nineties attending a rave!" Max went on, attracting more laughter.

"I tell you what I've gathered from seeing all these vendors here," one of the other people said, "is that we don't need any more tech solutions to fix what's wrong with our industry."

This attracted some murmurs of agreement.

"What we need," he went on, "is a magic wand."

Everyone burst out laughing. Josh nodded to Max as he had reached the correct floor, stepped out of the lift, and headed to the lounge with the beginnings of an idea forming in his head.

Chapter Twenty-five – The Mentor

Josh was pleased to see the lounge was empty so settled at an available desk to write down a few notes and add some elements to one of his mind maps. He knew he should probably try to relax to allow the thoughts to swirl around in his sub-conscious – hopefully in imitation of some kind of Small Hadron Collider such that two thoughts might collide and generate a spark of something new.

He also thought it was time he discussed things with his mentor.

Relaxing into the chair at the desk, he flicked open the connection that would allow them to speak.

"Hi Dad," he said, smiling in recognition as that familiar face appeared in front of him.

"Hello, son," his mentor replied, "I was just doing a spot of gardening when you rang. How are things?"

"All good," Josh replied, giving an overview of his current project and that he was currently in a hotel room in Las Vegas.

"Sin City, eh?" came the response, "think your mother and I spent some time there once. Mind you, it could have been Blackpool – I always get those two mixed up."

Josh chuckled at his dad's joke. He considered Blackpool – a holiday resort town in the north-west of England – to be a fun place to spend some time. But Vegas it was not.

"So go on," his dad went on, "what can I do for you this time?"

Over the last few years – in particular since starting his podcast – Josh had found himself increasingly turning to his dad for feedback and advice.

It was not that his dad had been especially well-traveled or had a huge range of experiences outside of what Josh himself had had but there was something about the kindly, intelligent, supportive way he responded to questions that always helped to nudge Josh along the right path to finding the solutions he was looking for.

Josh explained what he had been doing so far, stopping to allow his dad to interject with pertinent questions that helped to clarify Josh's thinking, ending by repeating the magic wand wisecrack that had been made in the elevator just recently.

Josh could see his dad thinking – he'd always had a habit of running his forefinger around his mouth when he was coming up with his best ideas so Josh allowed him to continue uninterrupted.

"Well, Josh," his dad said after a few moments, "I think your man in the lift was probably onto something."

Josh grinned – it would have been unthinkable for his dad to use the word elevator instead of its British version, 'lift'.

"Go on," Josh said.

"A magic wand. Hmm. We're all adults here, so I'm assuming neither of us believes there is such a thing as a real magic wand."

Josh nodded in agreement, but found himself wondering if he was all that sure about the truth of that statement.

"But what if there was something that was as close as possible to being a magic wand without actually being one?"

Josh pondered this for a moment.

"I think I see what you're getting at," he said. "Can you elaborate?"

"'Fraid not, son," his dad replied, "there's more gardening to be done. And I think the line's going a bit dodgy. Anyway, I'll see you next time. Cheerio."

And with that the connection was lost.

Josh always hoped he could spend more time on these chats with his dad but then, as he opened his eyes and saw the closed laptop on the desk in front of him, he also wished he could have spent more time with him when he was alive.

Puzzle solver extraordinaire he may be, but he had not yet worked out how to make a video call to heaven, outside of in his own mind.

Chapter Twenty-six – The Rare Disease Patient

Later that day, following a burst of activity that saw Josh developing his thoughts and coming up with something he was itching to explore further, Max had arranged for Josh to meet a rare disease patient. This would be someone he said would be able to provide a different perspective from what had been learned through talking with Elizabeth Bennett of the patient group.

Josh turned up at the pre-booked meeting room and greeted Max. "Hi Max, how have things been going for you today? Still catching up with people you haven't seen for a while?"

Max chuckled and responded, "yep, still bumping into people. Surprised that so many of them are still keen to talk to me, actually. But that could simply be they want some of that Alexander Wexford magic to rub off on them, too."

Josh smiled and asked who they would be seeing next.

"Well Black," Max responded, "this might surprise you, but the rare disease patient you'll be talking with is me."

Josh could not contain his surprise and looked at Max quizzically, Max laughing in response.

"Ha, thought that would be a bit of a shock to you," he said. "But yes, I am actually living with a rare condition, and have been for many years."

Josh was intrigued, and also realized he was concerned for the welfare of this man whom he now considered to be a friend.

Max obviously noticed Josh's expression and sought to reassure him. "Touching of you to care, Black – and I don't mean that in a sarcastic way, but it'll be some time before you see the back of me. Despite my condition likely being the eventual cause of my demise, it's currently under control. And I'm hoping to keep it that way for a good while yet."

Max went on to describe the nature of the rare disease he was living with, and how it was a genetically-inherited disorder affecting around 1 in 5,000 people.

"The two main definitions of rare disease," Max said, "are a condition that affects less than 1 in 2,000 people, or one that affects less than 200,000 people overall in the US. Broadly speaking, those two statistics reflect about the same percentage of the population either way."

Josh wanted to find out more but was apprehensive about prying too deeply until Max assured him it was fine and he was happy to discuss anything about his experience, especially when it related to patient recruitment.

"So is there a difference," Josh asked, "between the experience of someone living with a rare condition compared to someone living with, for example, diabetes?"

Max leaned back and nodded, thoughtfully.

"That's an interesting question, Black," he replied, "to which the most accurate answer would be 'I don't know'. The reason being that I don't have experience of living with diabetes so I can't really tell you. However, in the spirit of what you're getting at, I've obviously spoken with many people living with multiple conditions – both rare and non-rare – and I've concluded that, fundamentally, the experience is the same for the patient in either case.

"However, there can be vast differences in the way the industry behaves towards those of us living with rare conditions compared to people living with more common diseases. You mentioned diabetes, and that's certainly an area that gets a lot more attention than any rare disease. No surprise, of course, when you see that approximately one in eleven or twelve of the adult population actually has diabetes – so the potential for making money is obviously much greater.

And let's not forget that, outside of the profit potential, being able to make lives easier for that number of people is most definitely a worthy aim. So I have no problem with big pharma targeting the big headline conditions with their investigational treatments."

Max paused, allowing Josh to absorb this information – something Max knew Josh was apt to do.

"In the past there could often be something of a 'poor relation' effect," he went on, "when it came to looking at rare diseases. Over the last few years, though, and in particular with the rise in the number of biotech firms, there has been much more of a focus on rare disease within the industry. Such that even my own condition has multiple trials running at the moment for potential new treatments."

"And have you taken part in a trial yourself?" Josh asked.

"That's another interesting question, Black," Max replied, "and one that actually has quite an interesting answer. In truth, the whole reason I'm involved in this industry is due to the fact I originally took part in a clinical trial what must be around twenty years ago now. Matter of fact, it's how I met Alexander in the first place, with all that then resulted from that fortuitous happenstance."

Josh could tell from Max's more flowery language that he was warming to his theme.

"Actually highlights another area we should be thinking about," Max continued. "Those patients who are not members of advocacy groups or other types of support group. Back in the day I was a bit of a head in the sand person about my condition. The symptoms weren't showing yet, and – though I knew there was no escaping it as it's an inherited thing – I was trying to avoid much of anything to do with being ill.

So I was simply going about my life without considering myself to be a patient as indeed the vast majority of people do. Being defined by your condition is something that only a very small number of people are interested in. The rest of us simply want to get on with living our lives. Sure, if there was some kind of magic wand we could wave to make ourselves better, we'd all take it."

Josh made another mental note here – that magic wand image just kept coming up recently.

"But truth be told," Max went on, "in this rich tapestry where some of us might believe ourselves to be the center of the universe, the thought of attending group meetings to discuss our health with strangers is not something we pay much attention to."

"And yet you did take part in a trial, you said?" Josh asked.

"Well spotted, Black," Max replied, "I did indeed take part in a trial. And do you know how I found out about it?"

Josh shook his head.

"My sister told me," Max said. "Being imbued with a sense of fraternal love that I'm not sure I'll ever be able to fathom for myself, she was always on the look out for anything that might prove to be beneficial for my well-being – having avoided the genetic inheritance herself as we don't share the same father.

Interestingly, even though it's obvious that rare disease patients and their relatives are likely to be on social media and other websites – so promoting trials using those methods could be effective for rare diseases too – she came across an interview in a magazine with a rare disease patient who was discussing my very condition, and how he was taking part in a trial that was looking for additional volunteers. Shows the value of casting a wide net when it comes to looking for volunteers, Black. If my sister hadn't read that article because I wasn't involved with any type of patient group, I'd have never known about the trial.

Some of these patients – and even some doctors – can be considered 'influencers'. And I don't mean the type who might appear on the internet in a swimsuit, so developing a relationship with these types of people can be beneficial for disseminating information about trials. Quite a lot of people living with a rare disease, for instance, can become trusted voices for others with the same condition – which can help if you can get one on board to talk about what trial participation is like and how beneficial it can be for the community as a whole.

Fairly obviously, with a rare disease, there's a low number of patients to be able to target and often they have good communities and support groups in place already but, as I say, not everyone with a rare disease – or even a more common one – wants to be involved in that sort of thing.

And as we already know from our other conversations, the burden of participation can be a real turn-off. But even more than that, what we sometimes forget in this industry is that not everyone with a particular condition is actually interested in taking part in a clinical trial. Assessing the level of interest among the patient population might well be something we want to look at as being an essential ingredient for an effective solution.

On top of this, of course, there's the issue that, being rare, it's not all that common for primary care physicians to come across or be aware of them which can often lead to years of misdiagnosis before a correct diagnosis is made – something within the rare disease world they describe as 'looking for the horses, not the zebras'.

It's also the case that rare diseases can cross multiple specialisms, so patients are often frustrated that the specialists they see don't communicate with each other soon enough which could prevent delays and lead to a proper diagnosis much earlier."

Max went on to describe how the CRO operating the trial he had been on was a mid-size British firm called Awex, and how he had become so intrigued by the process he had sought out Alexander Wexford personally and contacted him to see if he could become involved with the company.

Wexford had been impressed by Max's ingenuity and enthusiasm so brought him in to shadow his own activities for a month before giving him his first job and sponsoring him through relevant academic studies that would help in his future career.

"But anyway, Black," Max said after an hour or so of discussion, "tell me what you've been working on so diligently while I've been schmoozing and glad-handing."

Chapter Twenty-seven – The Magic Wand Index

Josh collected his thoughts for a moment or two before outlining the idea he had come up with.

"Well, Max," he said, "it's funny you mentioned a magic wand earlier. The idea must have been sparked by that guy in the elevator earlier today then it's been brewing in my brain until I worked through the basic concept a few hours ago."

Max settled back in his chair, awaiting more on this new idea.

"It seems to me," Josh went on, "that there's no single solution – a magic wand, if you like – that will solve the problems of patient recruitment."

"Try telling that to Hank Davidson!" Max smirked.

Josh smiled, remembering how enthusiastic the patient recruitment solutions provider had been about his own firm's digital-first approach, and continued.

"Well, as we're all adults here," Josh continued, using his fingers to put quote marks around the word 'adults' which got a smile from Max, "we know there is no such thing as an actual magic wand. But maybe we can try to ensure that our solutions are as close to that as possible and, in order to get to that point, we'll need some method of measuring those solutions so we can improve the relevant elements of them as necessary."

Josh leant forward, resting his elbows on the desk and his chin in his hands then continued. "Which is where the Magic Wand Index comes in."

Max's eyes darted up and to the left as he sought to remember if he had heard this phrase before.

"I'll explain," Josh went on. "Each patient recruitment solution on offer has various elements within it that we can isolate and measure against the ideal. That is, we can look at the different components of what's being offered, then measure how close those components are to providing what we'd get if we had a real magic wand delivering the results.

"In the same way that Russ Johnson has identified the five stages of the patient recruitment process, with the Magic Wand Index I've identified the five elements of a solution that can be measured to determine if they're close to being magic, or closer to being meh."

Max listened intently, eager to hear what Josh had come up with.

"Firstly," Josh said, "the solution has to be relevant to what's being sought. So, for example, if somebody wants to bulk up their physique, a weight loss product would be meh, while a weight gain product will be magic.

Secondly, there has to be a perceived benefit so, to continue with the same example, if the extra bulk amounts to 1% of body mass, the benefit will be meh whereas if it's closer to 100%, the benefit will be perceived as being magic.

Thirdly, there has to be a worthwhile ROI. In our bulking product example, if the cost is $20,000 that will be perceived as meh, while a cost of $10 per month might be seen as magic.

Fourthly, the process needs to be simple to carry out. If there's a complicated set of instructions for taking a set number of tablets at specific times of day while only eating certain foodstuffs and having to do two hours of daily meditation, it will be viewed as meh while a once a week half hour workout that achieves the desired effect will be seen as being magic.

Fifth and finally, the results need to be achieved quickly. If it's going to take ten years to see any increase in bulk that will be seen as meh but if there are significant results within two weeks, that will be magic."

Josh paused to let Max ponder what he had been saying. He was unsure yet himself whether the Magic Wand Index was likely to be as useful a tool as he imagined it could be so was interested to hear Max's reaction.

"Black," Max began, stroking the side of his face as he sometimes did when about to make a pronouncement, "I think you might just well be onto something there."

Josh breathed a metaphorical sigh of relief, awaiting Max's next comments.

"So what you're saying is," Max continued, "we can use the Magic Wand Index as a tool to discover how effective a particular patient recruitment solution might be then seek to improve the elements that are closer to meh, and retain the elements that are closer to magic?"

Josh smiled. "You got it," he responded, "that's exactly how I think it would be able to be used and even the elements that are closer to being magic could potentially benefit from some refinements once we know where they sit on the scale."

"OK then," Max replied, "let's put it to the test. And while we're at it, why don't we see if we can overlay it on top of Russ's five stages."

Josh agreed that this would be a good idea, and added "and also look at it from the perspective of the various different stakeholders."

Max nodded, and Josh could tell he was becoming more excited.

"OK then," Max said, "Russ's first stage is to find the potential participants. Let's look at Hank's solution and view it through the lens of the Magic Wand Index."

"Sure, "Josh began. "Firstly, is a digital outreach approach relevant for finding people who might want to take part in trials?"

Max interrupted him. "Just a second, Black," he said, "what sort of scale are we going to use?"

They had a quick discussion about what they might use ranging from most magic to most meh – ranging from having Gandalf as the most magic to having a scripted reality TV show as the most meh, with various increments such as Harry Potter, Penn and Teller, daytime soaps and Saturday night gameshows in between before finally settling on a simple scale of 1-10, with 1 being meh and 10 being magic.

"OK," Josh resumed, "how magic or meh is a digital outreach approach for finding potential trial participants?"

"I think Hank would say 10," Max replied, "but I'd probably settle for a 7. Not everybody is on social media or other websites, after all."

Josh agreed and recorded the score of 7 in a notepad.

"Secondly," he went on, "does the digital approach deliver a perceived benefit to the people most interested in recruiting patients?"

"That's probably a 6 or a 7," Max replied. "Many sponsor firms don't trust digital outreach as a method, but are quite often convinced when they see it in practice."

Josh recorded the score of 6-7 and continued. "Thirdly, then, does that approach deliver a worthwhile ROI?"

"Another interesting one," Max replied. "Hank's firm primarily works on a pay-per-patient basis so with the sponsor agreeing to a set amount for each patient recruited, they'd obviously believe the ROI to be a good one, so probably an 8 if the results come in.

"On the other hand, some firms operate in an agency style where the sponsor simply pays a management fee and pass through costs for ad spend. This can work well, but can also lead to sponsors dishing out the moolah for low returns."

"So let's put this down as between 6 and 8," Josh said, before continuing. "Fourthly, is a digital outreach approach simple?"

"Again interesting," Max replied, "as we heard from Hank, there can often be something of a break in the process once the initial ads have been clicked on. Whether this is entirely the fault of the research sites I'm not sure, but it does involve some complication in that aspect. And there's often a learning curve on the part of the sites and others to get to grips with the backend system the vendors put in place."

"Just a 5 for this one, then?" Josh asked. Max agreed, so Josh went on. "And fifthly, how quick is this approach at delivering results?"

"Can be very quick indeed," Max replied. "I've seen some projects where the results start coming in from day one. Rare diseases might take longer though."

"So between 6 to 8 again," Josh said, then added up the total. "Between 30 and 35 for the digital outreach approach. Not exactly magic, but a long way from being meh."

"And if we look at the lowest scorer," Max said, reading Josh's notes, "we can see it's the simplicity of the process – in particular when it comes to booking the patients in for a screening visit – where the most improvement can be made which pretty much rings with everything we know to be true about that approach."

Max closed his eyes and thought for a moment.

"Black," he said, opening his eyes to stare directly at Josh and smile broadly, "I'm impressed. The Magic Wand Index might indeed be a highly effective tool for measuring the likely success of a particular patient recruitment solution. Not only suggesting whether it's worth pursuing in the first place, but also highlighting the aspects of the solution that should be looked at for improvement. Let's try it on another."

With that, Josh and Max continued for the next ninety minutes, analyzing various different solutions, and even specific pieces of software or individual activities, to test the validity of the Magic Wand Index as a tool for determining effectiveness.

Eventually, Max leaned back in his chair and said "this is all excellent stuff, Black. But unfortunately, simply having a tool to measure a solution's effectiveness – and, admittedly, that tool also being able to be used to make improvements – doesn't really provide an overall solution in itself."

Josh could only agree, but said he had something else in mind to bring to the party such that when he eventually presented his thoughts to Alexander Wexford, the whole should be greater than the sum of its parts.

They adjourned to the bar – the conference having ended for the day and the alcohol-fueled networking starting to get underway – and enjoyed the rest of the evening. As indeed they enjoyed the rest of the conference before heading back to England and a wrap-up meeting with Alexander Wexford.

Chapter Twenty-eight – Solving the Patient Recruitment Conundrum

Josh was not surprised that the same black Rolls-Royce with private registration plates was once again his mode of transport for the meeting with Alexander Wexford. Nor that Wexford's butler greeted him with the same warm formality as previously, and escorted him to the study where Wexford and Max were sitting waiting for him.

"Black, how wonderful to see you again. Been ages," joked Max, clapping Josh on the shoulder before enveloping him in a hug.

"And you, Max," Josh replied, then to Alexander Wexford, "Mr. Wexford."

Alexander Wexford unexpectedly also hugged Josh, the three of them momentarily locked in a slightly awkward embrace.

"Call me Alexander, Josh," Wexford said, "it's only people like Max here who prefer to use surnames. Something to do with one of those secret fraternities he went to in the States or something."

Max grinned and unlocked their embrace.

"So, Josh," Alexander said, gesturing for them all to sit down around a low table that was already adorned with several glasses, an open bottle of Pouilly-Fume, and one of champagne, "Max tells me you've solved the greatest problem facing the industry?"

"I'm not sure about that exactly," Josh replied, causing Alexander to sigh wistfully. "But I think my findings will reinforce what everyone probably already knows is the right way forward – though, for some reason, they simply aren't putting all that much effort into pursuing it."

"Pray tell," Alexander requested, pouring each of them a glass of wine.

Josh went on to outline the journey he and Max had been on, including descriptions of the various meetings they had had, and the sort of thinking Josh had brought to bear on the issues.

He went through an overview of the Magic Wand Index, delighting Alexander Wexford with the concept and how it could be used to assess how useful a proposed solution might be for recruiting and/or retaining patients.

"Makes me wish I was still in the game, old boy," Alexander said, his eyes suggesting he was seriously contemplating stepping back into the world of work for a moment before he took another sip of wine. "But, of course, I think it's probably best to leave that sort of thing to you younger guys to sort out for yourselves. And I couldn't possibly take on another job as I'm so busy here. What with the daily round of golf, the noon dip in the pool, the games of bridge with the boys…"

Max snorted a laugh at this point, causing Alexander to revise his statement.

"Well, OK," he said, "the games of poker with the boys. And all the holidays I have to take. For the good of my circulation. No, the world of clinical trials is better off without me."

"Though certainly better for your having been in it in the first place," Max interjected.

"No need to keep creeping up to me, Max," Alexander replied. "We've both sold our shares, you know."

They both laughed before Josh continued with his overview of where he thought the problems lay and what it might be possible to do about them.

Once he'd finished, Alexander and Max looked at each other and nodded.

"Josh Black, let me congratulate you," Alexander said, rising and offering his hand. Josh and Max both rose too, Josh shaking Alexander's hand who went on. "You've not only identified the key problems within the world of patient recruitment and retention, you've also pointed out a solution so obvious it's been staring everyone in the industry in the face for so long they've stopped noticing it."

"Rather like when you look in a mirror but don't see your own wrinkles?" Max asked.

"Speak for yourself, Max," Alexander replied. "I'm very proud of my own battle scars and notice every one of them. But anyway, our friend here has reinforced the view that many in the industry have expressed over the years, but sadly the will simply hasn't been there to incorporate it to any significant degree."

Alexander Wexford opened the champagne and raised a glass in toast to Josh and Max then bid them to sit down again as he had another suggestion in mind.

"Now then, Josh," he said, "let's see what we can do moving forwards."

He then outlined to Josh an idea for getting all the stakeholders involved in the clinical trials industry to support the central finding of Josh's puzzle-solving adventure. One aspect of this would involve incorporating the Magic Wand Index in future projects while the underlying theme was the one Josh had proposed as being the main issue preventing the progress that was necessary.

Josh did not need to think too hard before agreeing. He would be able to continue his podcasts, but his primary focus would be on actually delivering the change that was required rather than simply pointing it out. With Alexander Wexford's resources and Max's assistance, he was sure he would be able to have at least some small positive impact that could improve the world of patient recruitment and retention.

"Just one thing," Max said, as they toasted the success of their future endeavor, "what shall we call this venture?"

Josh smiled and started whistling a familiar tune. Alexander looked puzzled at first before Max burst out laughing and joined in. A few moments later, Alexander's butler was surprised when he came into the study cradling another bottle of champagne to find the three men engaged in a rendition of a song he had not heard for some years – Max singing the lead line, Josh whistling along, and Alexander tapping out the rhythm by clinking a champagne flute on a wine glass.

Chapter Twenty-nine – Let's Work Together

"Collaboration, not confrontation," Josh announced towards the end of his next podcast. "That's the only way to really solve the patient recruitment conundrum."

With Alexander Wexford's help, he and Max had spent the last two months setting up an organization dedicated to bringing the key stakeholders in clinical trials together in order to not only discuss their mutual issues, but ultimately work towards solving them.

Russ Johnson had been a brilliant sounding board, as had Hank Davidson, Elizabeth Bennett, Dan Kumar, Dr. Emma Fitzgerald and many other people Josh had met during his puzzle-solving journey.

He had also enjoyed several extremely useful 'conversations' with his mentor, and even managed to track down the guy in the Las Vegas elevator who had originally mentioned the 'magic wand'. It turned out the man had been there as a sales rep for a tech solutions provider but had subsequently become disillusioned with the product and walked away from it. Following several discussions, Josh had offered him a promotional role within the new organization.

"The Let's Work Together initiative," Josh announced to his listeners, "is designed to ultimately ensure better outcomes for all in the world of patient recruitment and retention for clinical trials. But more than that, it's based on making sure we all feel respected, encouraged, and welcomed within the industry.

The goal is for sponsors, CROs, research sites, patient groups, solutions providers, regulators, healthcare professionals, and individual patients alike to all be able to make their valuable contributions in a manner that makes them not only *feel* valued but actually *be* valued as an essential part of the whole.

Removing one of the bricks makes the whole tower fall down so let's keep all our bricks in place, and make sure we all work towards the same ends without the unnecessary pulling off course that sometimes characterizes this industry.

I hope you'll join me – and many others – as we push forward towards the best possible destination. Well, at least until someone discovers a real magic wand."

With that, Josh Black leaned back in his worn leather chair and reflected on how he had got here. He was delighted to have taken on Alexander Wexford's original challenge to uncover the flaws in the patient recruitment process and was even more keen to put those learnings into practice to try to achieve beneficial change within the industry.

He certainly was not underestimating the scale of what lay ahead, of course. A whole industry had ignored this basic principle of human endeavor for so long it had forgotten how essential it was for success. But he had hope that what he was doing was not going to be simply another talking shop, or lead to another load of guidelines and recommendations that nobody really paid much attention to in the real world.

'Let's work together', he thought, contemplating the hopefully bright and impactful future ahead. 'Let's work together indeed.'

Appendix

Josh's Notes and Mind Maps

Patient Recruitment Stakeholders

Research Sites
- responsible for dealing with patients, administering treatments, collecting data
- hospitals, academic centers, private clinics
- some are more competent than others

CRO (Contract Research Organization)
- manages the trial on behalf of the sponsor
- global, country specific, therapy area specialist, boutique
- some good, some bad

Sponsor
- funds the research and designs the trial
- pharma, biotech, medical device
- other – Investigator Initiated Studies

Patient Groups
- look after patients' interests
- advocacy, support, maybe charities (or not)

Patient Recruitment Vendors
- recruit patients into trials for a fee
- tech solutions, digital ads, traditional ads, community outreach, doctor outreach, databases, DCT solutions

Patients
- trial volunteers
- qualify for trial based on condition and usually location (proximity to research site)

Regulators
- set the rules governing how trials are conducted
- government agencies, Institutional Review Board (IRB) or Ethics Committee (EC)

Patient Recruitment Stakeholders

Sponsor — Funds the research
- Biotech
- Big Pharma
- Other - IIS
- Medical devices

CRO — Manage/Operate Trial on Sponsors behalf
- Global
- Specialist
- Country Specific
- Boutique

Research Sites — Sees Patients & administers trial treatment
- Hospitals
- Academic Institutions
- Private Clinics

Regulators — Set the Rules governing trials
- Ethics Committee / IRB
- Government Agencies

Patient Groups — Look after Patient Interests
- Support Groups
- Charities
- Advocacy Groups

Patients
- Location
- Condition
- Trial Volunteers
- DCT

Solutions Providers/Vendors — Recruit Patients into trials for a fee
- Patient Databases
- Tech Solutions
- Doctor Outreach
- Digital Ads
- Traditional Ads
- Community Outreach

Trial Participation

Patient Journey
- find out about trial, learn more, apply – may be uncontactable
- screening, qualifying via Inclusion/Exclusion (I/E) criteria – may not qualify
- consent (or not)
- randomization – placebo or active treatment
- site visits – may be 'lost to follow up' (drop out of trial)
- ongoing participation – retention on the trial

Burden of Participation
- possibly intrusive procedures
- multiple site visits
- burden of condition may make things worse
- time spent on site visits
- cost of travel, plus lost cost of attending visits
- expenses reimbursement?

Patient journey

- Finds out about trial
- Learns more
- Applies to take part
  - Not contactable
  - Screening
    - Not qualify
    - Qualify
      - Doesn't consent
    - Inclusion/Exclusion Criteria
    - Consents to take part
      - Randomization
        - Active treatment
        - Placebo
        - Research site visits
          - Lost to follow-up
          - Ongoing Participation
          - Retention of patient on trial
- Trial Participation
  - Burden of Participation
    - Intrusive procedures?
    - Multiple Visits
    - Travel
    - Cost
    - Expenses?
    - Time
  - Burden of Condition

Research Sites

Patient Interaction
- friendly, warm, mutual respect
- ongoing communication (not always good – unanswered calls) – birthday and thank you cards go down well

Trial Software
- difficult to keep track of multiple logins
- not especially user-friendly
- different one for each trial/vendor
- standardized systems to make life easier?

Site Involvement in Trial Design
- feedback from people 'on the ground'
- day to day trial operations – should provide good intel re: recruitment and retention

Central Ad Campaigns
- not usually very good ('forced' on the site by sponsor/CRO)
- can be a waste of time with patients not fitting I/E criteria
- Site's Own Ad Campaigns
- difficult process to get funds from sponsor (feel like 'begging')
- most sites not have own funds to manage (in significant amounts)

Inclusion/Exclusion (I/E) Criteria
- looking for 'unicorns'
- amount of criteria has increased and become more strict
- looking for superbeings with no co-morbidities

Payments to Sites
- bottom rung of the clinical trials ladder
- fair market value = how fair is it?

Research Sites

- **Trial design**
  - 'On the ground' feedback
  - Site Involvement
- **Central Ad Campaigns**
  - Not very good
- **Own Ad Campaigns**
  - Beg for Funds
- **Inclusion / Exclusion Criteria**
  - Unicorns
  - Super beings
- **Payments to sites**
  - Fair Market Value?
- **Patient interaction**
  - Friendly
  - Mutual Respect
  - Ongoing Communication
  - Unanswered Calls
- **Trial Software**
  - Multiple versions
  - Standardization?

Contract Research Organizations (CROs)

Site Selection & Feasibility
- experience
- medical infrastructure
- access to relevant patient populations

Other Connections
- patient groups
- physician networks

Patient Recruitment Vendors
- transparency and visibility an issue
- not always deliver what promise

Research Site Relationship
- sites don't always play ball
- can be too busy to respond in a timely manner

Sponsor Relationship
- procurement dept interaction, not clinical operations
- bid 'defense' – automatically puts the relationship into adversarial mode

Internal Communications
- silos between departments at the big CROs
- maybe the smaller CROs don't have silos

CROs

- **Patient Recruitment Vendors**
  - Transparency & visibility
  - Not always deliver
- **Research Sites**
  - Not always play ball
  - Too busy to respond
- **Sponsors**
  - Procurement Department
    - Not Clin ops
  - Bid 'Defense'
    - Combative
- **Physicians networks**
- **Site selection & feasibility**
  - Medical Infrastructure
  - Access to Patients
  - Experience
- **Patient Groups**
- **Internal Silos**
- **Boutique maybe not**

Patient Advocacy Groups

Environment
- hub for empowerment, support and advocacy
- resource library
- quiet room

Route to PAG Involvement
- family member (or self)
- likeminded community

What they Provide
- supportive community
- resources
- a voice for patients

Patient Database
- guarded against profiteering
- should be for improving treatments and quality of life
- collaborative partnerships with sponsors

Patient Involvement
- every stage of trial process from protocol design on
- patients embedded in the research teams
- build trust between patient and research community
- CROs should involved groups earlier in the process
- requires effective feedback loops

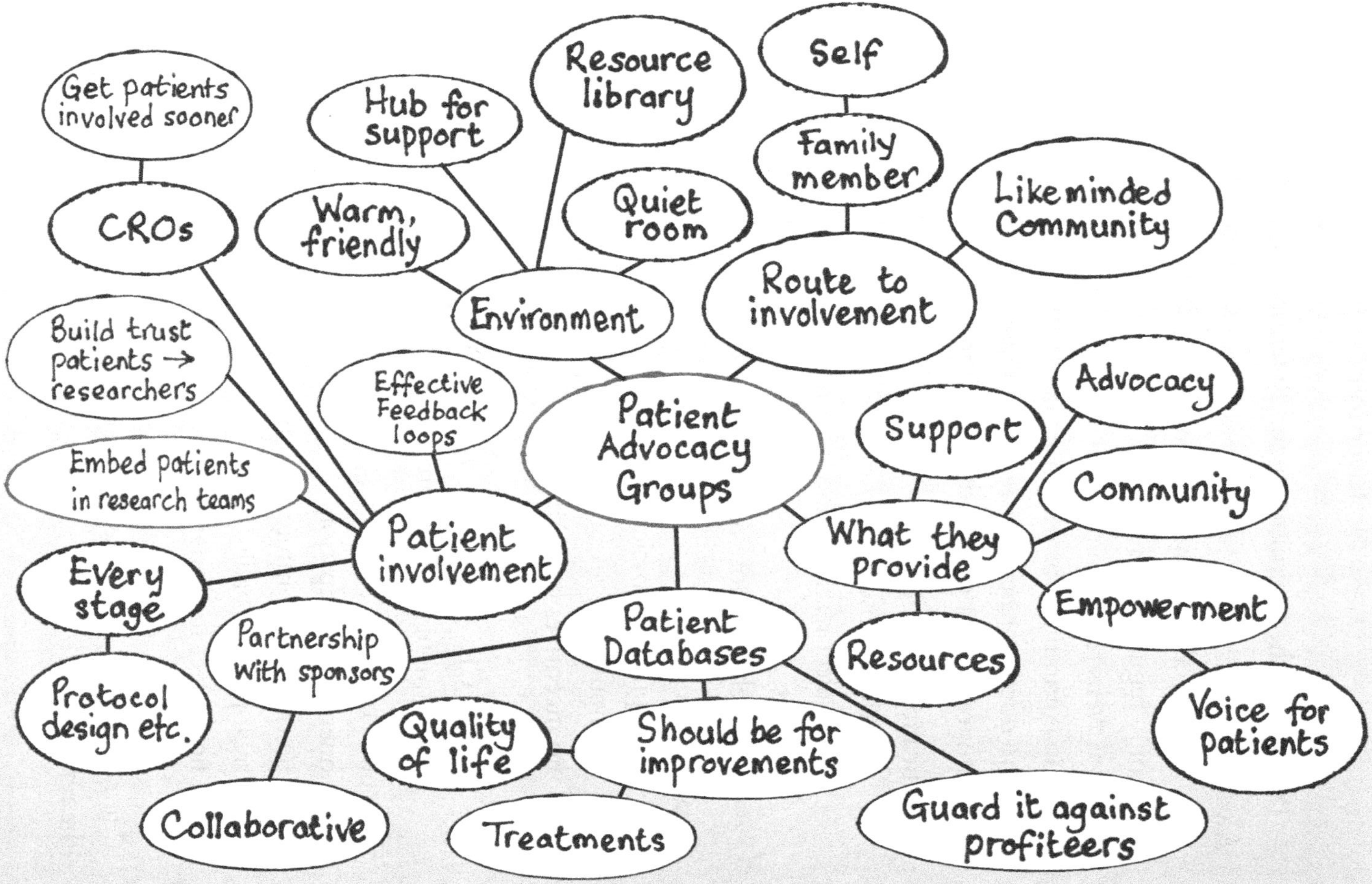

Inversion

(Setting up the Recruitment and Retention Process to Fail *)

Awareness
- nobody able to find out about the trial
- only regulatory presence
- no website or promotional materials
- no community or patient group outreach
- no doctor or health care professional (HCP) outreach
- no long-term relationship building

Qualification and Eligibility
- so strict almost nobody qualifies
- only select research sites with no or very few eligible patients
- only select remote research sites that are difficult to access

Trial Design
- no input from patients
- no input from research sites
- no incentives for taking part – either patients or anyone else
- global CRO to operate, without assistance from patient recruitment solutions providers

Patient Burden
- onerous participation
- no ongoing communication
- treat patients badly
- no respect for patient involvement

(* a mental model exercise in order to actually do the opposite in the real project)

Inversion: How to set up the project to fail

- **Awareness**
  - No promo
    - Only regulatory presence
    - No website
  - No outreach
    - Doctors/HCPs
    - Patient groups
    - Community groups
  - No relationship building
- **Qualification & eligibility**
  - Only research sites with no patients
    - Remote, difficult to access
  - Extremely strict I/E criteria
- **Trial design**
  - No input
    - Research sites
    - Patients
  - Global CRO
    - No patient recruitment vendors
    - No incentives
- **Patient burden**
  - Onerous participation
  - No ongoing communication
  - Treat patients
    - Badly
    - No respect

Big Pharma

Patient Involvement in Trial Design
- regulatory bodies
- historical factors
- patient-centricity

Eligibility Criteria
- balance between rigor and wide range of people
- engaging with patient groups, research sites, patients
- leveraging technology
- investigative treatments need to meet efficacy requirements
- cost of failed studies
- ongoing studies 'in market'
- Investigator Initiated Trials

Relationships
- CROs, sites, and vendors – lack of visibility and transparency
- overestimates of recruitment capabilities
- CRO A team, B team approach
- Internal silos
- Sales teams & MSLs – trial awareness
- preferred supplier status – any actual preference?

Global Nature of Trials
- cultural differences
- language issues
- I/E criteria issues

Patient Populations
- diversity, equity, inclusion
- ethnicity, gender, sexual orientation, socio-economic status

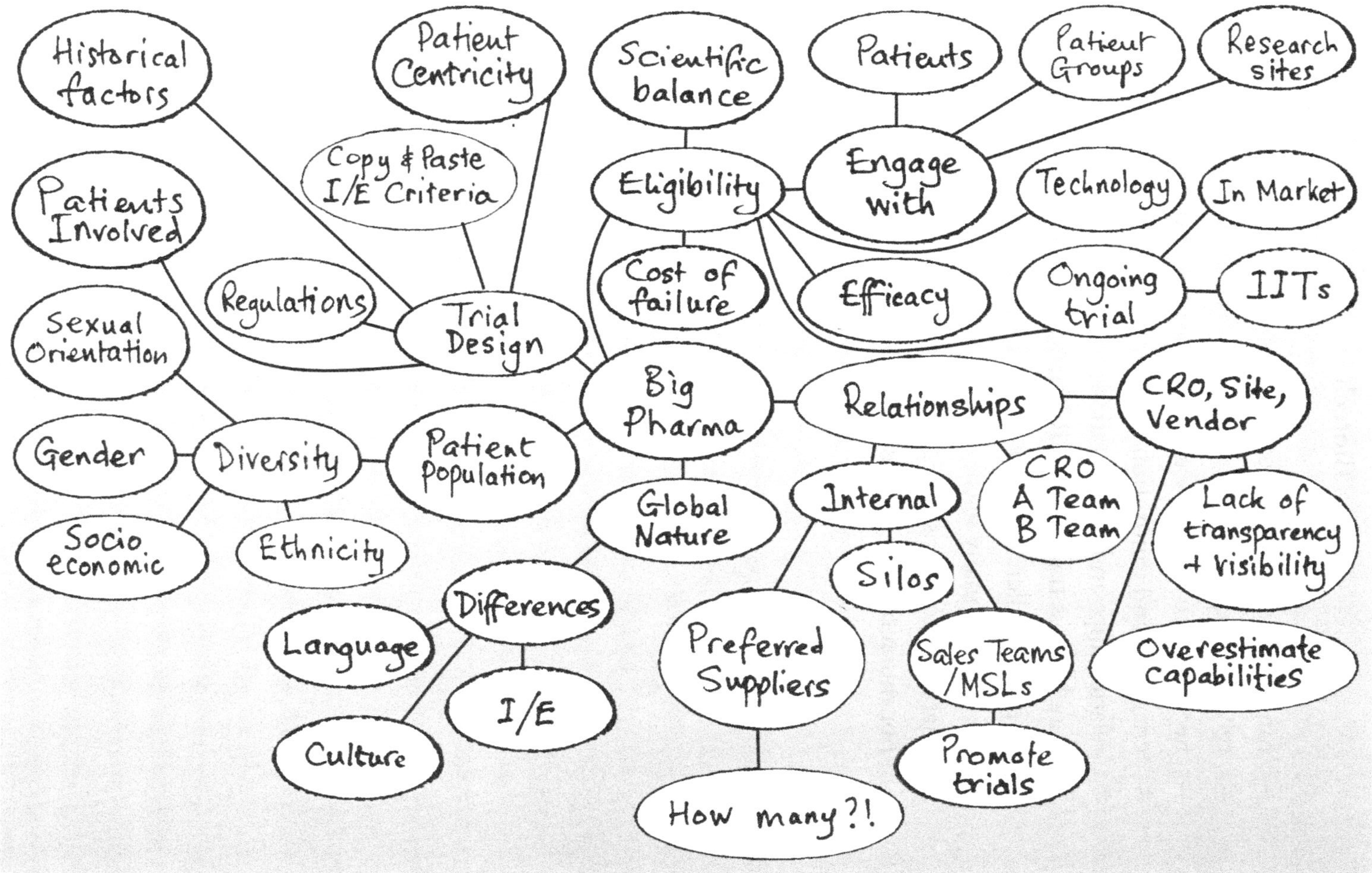
Historical factors
Patient Centricity
Copy & Paste I/E Criteria
Scientific balance
Patients
Patient Groups
Research sites
Patients Involved
Eligibility
Engage with
Technology
In Market
Regulations
Trial Design
Cost of failure
Efficacy
Ongoing trial
IITs
Sexual Orientation
Big Pharma
Relationships
CRO, Site, Vendor
Gender
Diversity
Patient Population
CRO A Team B Team
Internal
Socio economic
Ethnicity
Global Nature
Lack of transparency + visibility
Silos
Differences
Language
Preferred Suppliers
Sales Teams /MSLs
Overestimate capabilities
I/E
Culture
Promote trials
How many?!

Biotech

- funding and resources less than big pharma
- rely on investors
- need trials to work at each stage for more funding
- creativity and innovation
- relationships and collaborations
- may by-pass traditional CRO arrangement
- or use a smaller, boutique CRO
- CEO wears many hats
- enables quick decisions
- not much time to research solutions

Biotech

- **Funding & Resources**
  - Rely on Investors
  - Less than Big Pharma
  - Different stages of trial
    - Success = more funds
- **Creativity**
- **Relationships + Collaborating**
  - Innovation
    - Boutique CRO
  - By-pass Traditional CRO
- **Staff wear many hats**
  - Quick decisions
  - Not much time to research solutions

Ethics Committee (EC) / Institutional Review Board (IRB)

Responsibilities
- safeguarding patients rights and welfare
- evaluate scientific merit, ethical considerations, risks
- patient-centricity
- diversity and inclusion
- protect patients – investigative treatments are unproven so could be harmful

Board members
- experienced and level of expertise
- range of backgrounds – medical, researchers, patients etc.
- forthcoming mandated patients and members of public

Review Materials
- lots of information and detail – quite a burden to review
- informed consent – direct adverts are first stage of process
- complex issues of expanded access of non-approved treatments

Trial Participants
- payments for taking part?
- data privacy issues

EC/IRB

- **Board Members**
  - Experienced
  - Diversity & Inclusion
  - Range of backgrounds
    - Medical
    - Research
    - Patients
    - Public
    - Mandated
    - Expert
- **Responsibilities**
  - Merits of trial
    - Patient-Centricity
    - Ethical
    - Risk
    - Scientific
    - Safeguard Patients
      - Investigative Treatments
      - Could be harmful
  - Trial Participants
    - Payments?
    - Data Privacy
  - Review Materials
    - Informed Consent
      - Adverts
    - Lots of info
    - Expanded access
    - Complex

Patient Recruitment Vendor – Digital Outreach

Online Platforms
- Facebook Ads (majority)
- targeted campaigns
- personalized messaging
- often 60%+ trial participants
- data-driven strategies
- ongoing optimization

Landing Page
- user friendly
- pre-screening
- contact details
- ethical guidelines
- follow-up calls
- arrange research site visit

Payment Models
- agency style
- pay per lead
- pay per patient

Research Sites
- delays and inefficiencies arranging site visits
- utilize existing systems for booking visits
- I/E criteria
- Locations

Industry Reputation
- 'guinea pig' comments
- improvement would help recruitment

Digital Outreach

- **Online Platforms**
  - Data-driven strategies
  - Ongoing Optimisation
  - Messaging
  - Facebook Ads
    - 60%+ Trial participants
    - 'Guinea Pig' Comments
  - Targeted
- **Landing Page**
  - User Friendly
  - Pre-Screen
  - Contact
    - Follow-up
    - Site Visit
  - Ethics guidelines
  - Platform guidelines
- **Research Sites**
  - I/E Criteria
  - Locations
  - Delays in Booking Visit
  - Utilise existing systems
- **Industry**
  - Improve Reputation
- **Payment Models**
  - Pay per Patient
  - Pay Per Lead
  - Agency

Decentralized Trials (DCTs)

Trial Participation
- not have to attend research site
- tech includes digital platforms, wearables, telemedicine
- eConsent, ePRO
- home visits
- online visits
- non-site visits
- mobile research sites
- primary care providers
- retail pharmacies

Fundamentals
- innovative ways and processes
- not just tech
- choice
- flexibility
- options
- tech + human element

Mind Map: Trial Participation

Trial Participation connects to:
- Doctor visits
- Retail Pharmacies
- Mobile Sites
- On-line Visits
- Non-Site Visits
- Home visits
- Tech
- DCTs

Tech connects to:
- Telemedicine
- ePro
- Wearables
- Digital Platforms
- eConsent

DCTs connects to:
- Not have to attend site
- Innovative ways and processes
- Fundamentals

Innovative ways and processes connects to:
- Not just Tech

Fundamentals connects to:
- Choice
- Flexibility
- Options
- Tech + Human element

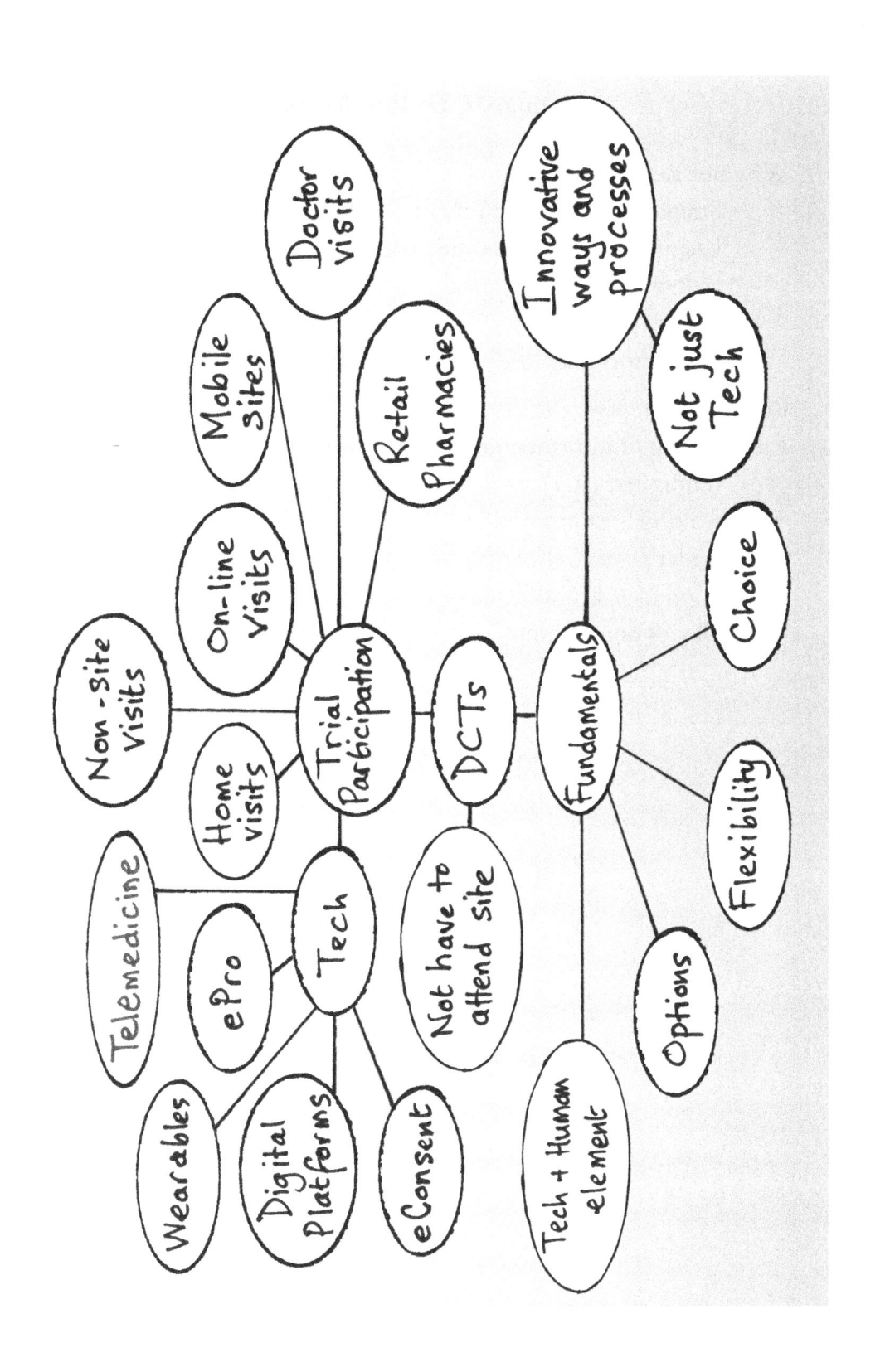

Primary Care Physicians

Why not Refer Patients?
- limited time in appointments
- keeping up with trials and criteria
- lack of awareness of suitable trials
- risks to patients
- US doctors may lose patient to other provider

Referral Attempts
- timing of information – patient overwhelmed by diagnosis (reminders later)
- waiting area promotions – limited success with TV or leaflet promo
- good idea, but difficult to see things changing in current way of doing things

Mind Map

- **Primary Care Physicians**
  - **Limited Time**
    - For keeping up with info
    - In appointments
  - **Lack of awareness**
  - **Why not refer?**
    - Risk to patients
    - Risk to Doctor
      - US – Patient may switch
  - **Referral Attempts**
    - **Timing Issue**
      - Patient Overwhelmed
        - Not taken details
        - Remind later
    - **Good Idea**
      - Unlikely to improve anytime soon
    - **Waiting area promo**
      - Leaflets
      - TV
      - Limited Success

Rare Disease Patients

Rare Disease Definitions
- affects less than 1 in 2,000 people
- affects less than 200,000 people in the US
- both the above are approx. the same in terms of patient populations

Experience
- rare and non-rare patients have fundamentally same experiences of conditions
- industry treats them differently
- long time for diagnosis
- doctors looking for 'horses' not 'zebras'
- specialists not consult with each other
- patients not define themselves as their condition (or conditions)

Recruiting Patients
- by nature of being rare are small numbers of people
- influencers can promote trials
- potentially low returns so industry not traditionally interested
- biotechs and others targeting rare disease more commonly now
- rare disease patients don't live in a vacuum – social media can be useful

Rare Disease Patients

Definition
- <1 in 2,000 People
- Approx. same total population
- <200,000 People in US

Experience
- Rare & non-rare fundamentally same
- Industry treats differently
- Long time for diagnosis
  - Horses not zebras
- Specialists not consult each other
- Patients are NOT their condition

Recruiting Patients
- Social Media
- Biotechs and others now targetting rare disease
- Influencers
- Rare = Small number of People
- Potentially low ROI for industry

Other Factors and Solutions

Main Issues
- awareness – lack of awareness
- access – lack of access

Recruitment Process
- finding patients
- engaging with them
- qualifying them against I/E criteria
- consenting – having the patients consent to participate
- retaining them on the trial
- Industry Conferences
- can come away thinking all is fine (preaching to the converted)
- can soon forget what have learned once get back into daily routine

Other Types of Trial
- observational
- apps, non-clinical trials

Other Solutions
- site networks (utilize mutual databases of potential patients)
- swift follow-up qualification by medically-trained people
- translating materials into non-English languages (can also help in English-speaking areas)
- influencers, Key Opinion Leaders (KOLs)
- tech for quicker chart review process (e.g. AI)
- patient databases
- trial 'marketplaces' – online platforms for participants to research potential trials
- patient retention gifts
- gamification of e.g, ePRO
- concierge service for patient travel and accommodation
- medical records
- duplicate virtual patients

Other factors & Solutions

- **Industry Conferences**
  - Observational
  - Apps, non-clinical
  - Other types of trial
  - Forget when back day to day
  - Preaching to converted

- **Site networks**
  - Utilize mutual DBs
  - Medically qualified
  - Influencers & KOLs

- **Swift follow-up**
  - Non-English translation
    - Also for English speaking regions

- **Main issues**
  - Lack of access
  - Lack of awareness
  - Recruitment Process
    - Finding
    - Engaging
    - Qualifying
    - Consenting
    - Retaining

- **Medical records**
  - Duplicate virtual Patients

- **Patient retention gifts**
  - Concierge Service

- **Quicker chart review**
  - AI

- **Patient DBs**
  - Trial Marketplaces

- **Gamification**
  - e.g. ePRO

Magic Wand Index

Measuring the Value of a Solution
- relevance to the desired outcome
- perceived benefit
- worthwhile ROI
- simplicity of implementation
- speed of results

Measurement Scale
- most magic = 10
- most 'meh' = 1
- highlights areas that may need improvement

Practical Applications
- patient recruitment solutions
- drill down to individual elements
- wider application for any type of solution

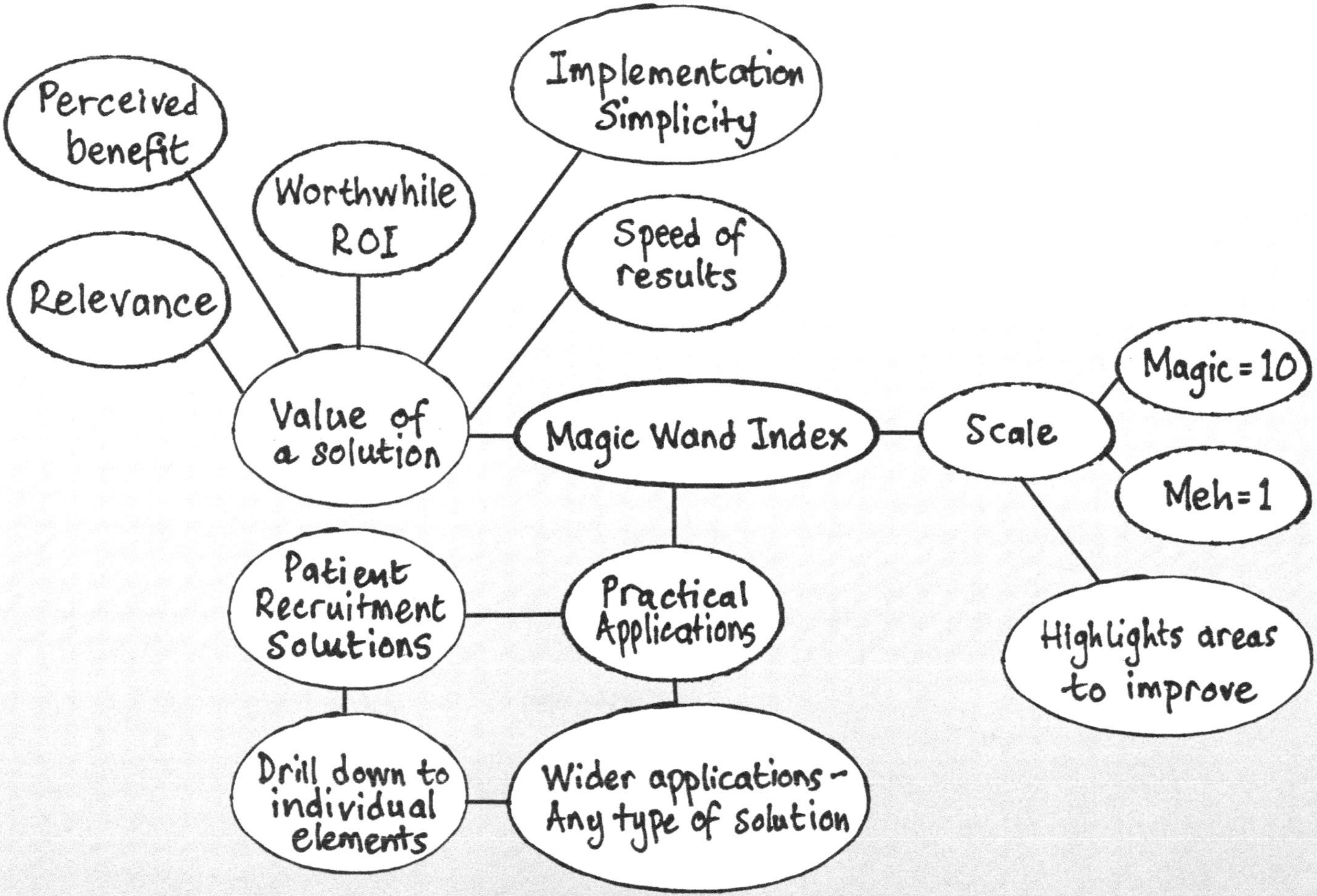
Magic Wand Index
Value of a solution
Perceived benefit
Relevance
Worthwhile ROI
Implementation Simplicity
Speed of results
Scale
Magic = 10
Meh = 1
Highlights areas to improve
Practical Applications
Patient Recruitment Solutions
Drill down to individual elements
Wider applications - Any type of solution

Acknowledgments

My thanks to the many dedicated professionals I've learned so much from over the years I've been working in patient recruitment and retention.

For this project in particular I wish to thank everyone who cast an eye over some of the contents and provided feedback prior to publication, including: Alex Billington, Amy Cavers, Andreas Beust, Bert Hartog, Carole Scrafton, Craig Lipset, Daniel Fox, Elizabeth Weeks-Rowe, Jason Gubb, Robert Goldman, Robert Joyce, Seth Rotberg, Wes Michael.

Your input has helped to make this book better. Any errors and omissions that remain are, of course, all my own.

For the creation of the book itself, I've had assistance with editing, illustrating, publishing formatting, and cover design. Respectively: Alison Parkin, Jan White, Joan Akwue, and Liam Beale. Thanks also to each of you.

For readers – if you like the book, please leave a positive review on Amazon.

If you didn't like it, please let me know directly via my website at RossJackson.com. (Indeed, you can let me know directly if you did like it, too.)

And thanks to you for reading!

About the Author

Ross Jackson is a patient recruitment specialist, based in Manchester, England.

He's the author of the Amazon best-selling book 'Patient Recruitment for Clinical Trials using Facebook Ads' (leading to his being described as 'the Godfather of social media patient recruitment') and has advised and consulted on over a hundred successful patient recruitment projects.

Having started out with digital marketing in 1998, Ross quickly developed a specialism in the healthcare niche, evolving into a focus on clinical trials and the problems of patient recruitment and retention.

Over the years Ross has branched out from the purely digital, and now operates in an advisory capacity helping sponsors, CROs, sites, solutions providers, and others in the industry to improve their patient recruitment and retention capabilities.

RossJackson.com

LinkedIn.com/in/RossJacksonConsulting

Made in the USA
Middletown, DE
07 January 2024

47195697R00109